WORKING WITH CLEFT PALATE

WORKING WITH CLEFT PALATE

JACKIE STENGELHOFEN

WP
WINSLOW PRESS
Telford Road, Bicester, Oxon OX6 0TS
Telephone: Bicester (0869) 244644

First published in 1990 by
Winslow Press, Telford Road, Bicester, Oxon OX6 0TS

Phototypeset by Gecko Limited, Bicester, Oxon

02-693/Printed in Great Britain by Hobbs the Printers, Southampton

British Library Cataloguing in Publication Data
Stengelhofen, Jackie
Working with cleft palate
1. Man. Cleft palate. Therapy
I. Title
617. 522506

ISBN 0–86388–079–7

CONTENTS

FOREWORD
vii

ACKNOWLEDGEMENTS
viii

INTRODUCTION
ix

CHAPTER 1
A REVIEW OF THE PHYSICAL FACTORS IN CLEFT LIP & PALATE
1

CHAPTER 2
THE NATURE OF THE SPEECH DIFFICULTIES
15

CHAPTER 3
ASSESSMENT OF THE SPEECH MECHANISM
25

CHAPTER 4
HOW CAN THE TEAM HELP?
39

CHAPTER 5
PATTERNS OF SPEECH THERAPY PROVISION
51

CHAPTER 6
GENERAL PRINCIPLES OF INTERVENTION
59

CHAPTER 7
WORKING WITH BABIES & YOUNG CHILDREN
63

CHAPTER 8
TREATMENT PROCEDURES FOR SPEECH
75

CHAPTER 9
INTRODUCTION TO INSTRUMENTATION
91

CHAPTER 10
CASE EXAMPLES
101

APPENDIX I
ORO-FACIAL EXAMINATION
112

APPENDIX II
DIAGNOSTIC RATING CHECKLIST
114

APPENDIX III
USEFUL ADDRESSES
115

BIBLIOGRAPHY
116

Jackie Stengelhofen

Jackie Stengelhofen has been working in the specialist field of cleft palate for the past 25 years. She first became interested in this area while working at the Queen Victoria Hospital, East Grinstead. This interest was pursued through her clinical and teaching involvement at the Dental Hospital and School, University of Birmingham.

From 1972 to 1988 she was Head of the School of Speech Therapy, Birmingham Polytechnic, and was responsible for developing the four-year honours degree course there. Throughout her career in teaching she has maintained her clinical work, specialising in speech problems resulting from maxillo-facial and palatoglossal problems.

Currently, she is developing courses for clinical teachers for a range of health care professionals. Her wide experience in matters of course development led to her recent invitation from the University of Zimbabwe to advise on the setting-up of a speech therapy degree.

Her extensive experience as both a clinician and a teacher has enabled her to write a book which is a welcome addition to the Winslow Press *Working with . . .* series, and one which every clinician will want to have on their shelf for immediate reference and for a wealth of treatment guidelines.

Foreword

The author skilfully distils her many years of clinical experience to produce a book primarily aimed at the community-based speech therapist who works only occasionally with children with cleft lip and/or palate.

Much of the existing literature is designed for the hospital-based specialist speech therapist and is mainly theoretical in nature, with frequent emphasis on assessment. Although these issues are of vital importance and interest, the concern of the community-based therapist is to know how to help their particular patient's speech problems. As the author rightly points out, many therapists, when faced with a child with a cleft lip and/or palate, feel particularly inadequate. Here, however, is a manual designed specifically as a practical guide for the clinician. This handbook encourages the therapist to consider the total child, and provides a comprehensive and systematic framework in which the therapist can consider all the possible aetiological factors in the communication disorder. By pointing out the importance of the interaction of the vocal tract, therapists are encouraged not to overlook phonation, an often neglected area with these patients. Perhaps the greatest strength of *Working with Cleft Palate* lies in the large collection of practical therapeutic ideas, some of which have been drawn from a range of specialist texts not usually found on the clinic shelves of the local health centre. Specialist speech therapists will find this aspect of the manual particularly useful, too.

A unique and valuable achievement of this book is to demonstrate the position of the community-based therapist in the large team of professionals responsible for a patient. In effect the therapist temporarily joins the hospital team, often providing unique and helpful information based on frequent and close contact with the patient and the patient's family. This book will give community-based therapists confidence and encouragement to recognise and fulfil their role in this team. This in turn will help prevent the creation of a divide between the hospital and the community.

Working with Cleft Palate will also be invaluable for students and in the training of speech therapy assistants, not only in the West but also in the developing world. It most usefully fills a gap in the literature.

Debbie Sell
Specialist Speech Therapist
London, 1990

ACKNOWLEDGEMENTS

The people I need to thank for help in the preparation of this book are too numerous to name individually. However I would like to thank in particular those individuals who gave me very specific comments and suggestions which helped me to get the draft stage into a comprehensible form: Charles Shute, of Birmingham Polytechnic; Kate Sweeny, of Booth's Hall Children's Hospital, Manchester; Cheryl Yeates, of the Queen Victoria Hospital, East Grinstead.

I would also like to give special thanks to the cohorts of fourth-year speech therapy students who graduated from Birmingham Polytechnic in 1989 and 1990, who read some draft chapters and provided honest and most constructive criticism.

Special thanks also to Val Dinning, not only for constant support, but also for providing the line drawings in Chapters 1, 3 and 4 and for reading the manuscript.

Thanks are due to many speech therapy colleagues, with whom I have been able to discuss cases and so gain a better understanding of many of the problems faced by clinicians in working with individuals with cleft lip and palate. Thanks also to many colleagues in other fields with whom I have worked, in particular to those in the Queen Victoria Hospital, East Grinstead and The Dental Hospital, Birmingham. My work with them has enhanced my understanding of the total management of cases and enabled me to experience the immense value of teamwork.

Finally gratitude is expressed to the many children and adults with whom I have had the privilege of working, without whom the preparation of this book would not have been possible.

INTRODUCTION

Working with Cleft Palate is for all clinicians and students who work or may work with cleft lip and/or palate patients. For the community-based clinician who has only occasional contact, as for the specialist clinician seeing patients on a regular basis, the book contains accessible and wide-ranging information on all aspects of assessment, management, intervention and treatment.

Chapter 1 offers an overview of the many physical factors which need to be considered in treatment, with line drawings augmenting the text. *Chapter 2* looks at the nature of speech difficulties and serves as a reminder of the essential concepts as preparation for practice.

With comprehensive, easy-to-read tables, *Chapter 3* details assessment procedures essential to the accurate evaluation of all aspects of the speech mechanism.

The team approach and the contribution of individual team members are considered in detail in *Chapter 4*, while patterns of provision discussed in *Chapter 5* encourage the reader to consider the prognosis, look at when intervention should begin and evaluate available provision — with a discussion of group versus individual treatment.

Chapter 6 offers much-needed information and general principles with regard to intervention. With specific reference to work with babies and young children, *Chapter 7* gives the reader a wealth of suggestions and practical ideas for intervention. In *Chapter 8* flow charts and tables supplement the text, which, once again, is positively practical in its approach to the treatment of insufficient nasality, excess nasality, dysphonia and articulation.

Chapter 9 offers an introduction to and explanation of available instrumentation and the final chapter records succinct case history examples to highlight treatment procedures across the age range, from young child to adult, which include assessment, case outlines, examination of the speech mechanism, intervention plans, therapy aims and methods.

The appendices contain an essential oro-facial examination form and a diagnostic rating checklist. Addresses of associations of particular relevance to readers are also included.

CHAPTER 1
A REVIEW OF THE PHYSICAL FACTORS IN CLEFT LIP & PALATE

The Necessary Skills and Knowledge / *2*

The Incidence of Cleft Lip and Palate / *3*

Types of Cleft and Consequences for Communication / *3*

- Cleft of Lip and Alveolus / *3*
- Clefts of the Hard and Soft Palate / *5*
- Complete Clefts / *7*

Delayed Surgery / *8*

Congenital Problems Affecting Velopharyngeal Function / *8*

Speech Problems After Adenoidectomy / *9*

Factors Which Have a Major Influence on the Development of Communication / *9*

- Hearing Impairment / *9*
- Dental Malocclusion / *10*
- Oro-nasal Fistula / *11*

Is Acceptable Speech Likely to Develop After Surgery? / *12*

CHAPTER 1
A REVIEW OF THE PHYSICAL FACTORS IN CLEFT LIP & PALATE

The Necessary Skills and Knowledge

Clinicians working with cleft palate cases appear to hold widely differing views about the complexity of treating communication problems associated with this condition. Some view it as a straightforward area, while others lack confidence and appear almost unable to start on the management because they believe that they do not have the prerequisite knowledge and skills. Clinicians who work routinely in a hospital or community setting carry only a very small number of cleft palate cases and it is therefore understandable that they feel uncertain as to how to proceed. In developing countries, where advanced surgery may not be available, clinicians may encounter different problems, for which they feel unprepared (**Sell & Woodard**, 1987). Clinicians in all situations should be reassured that they are already equipped with many of the generic skills which are relevant to working with individuals who have cleft lip and palate:

- Interpersonal skills;
- Observational skills;
- Skills to elicit speech and language data;
- Skills to analyse speech and language data;
- Skills to design intervention programmes;
- Skills to carry out remedial procedures.

Generic skills do not provide all the answers, however, as there are a number of factors which are of particular significance to the management of these cases. These include:

- The original condition, and the possible consequences;
- The types of operations and their appropriateness to the conditions;
- The functioning of the vocal tract;
- The impact of the original condition on:
  - phonation,
  - resonance,
  - articulation,
  - phonetic levels of speech;
- The role of the team and the speech clinician's function within it;
- The appropriateness of various types of intervention to the remediation process;
- The secondary problems and their relationship to communication;
- The availability and use of instrumental procedures;
- The problems presented in cases of unrepaired clefts.

This handbook is designed as a reference and practical guide for the clinicians and will address the points listed above. It is not intended to replace the essential, more detailed theoretical study, in such texts as **Bzoch** (1979); **Cooper *et al*** (1979); **Edwards & Watson** (1980); **Fletcher** (1972); **McWilliams *et al*** (1984) and **Stengelhofen** (1989).

The Incidence of Cleft Lip and Palate

The incidence of cleft lip and/or palate in the developed world is one in every 700 live births. The distribution of cleft lip and/or palate is generally reported as follows:

LIP ONLY	20%
PALATE ONLY	20%
LIP AND PALATE	60%

The palate-only group is the only group to have a higher incidence in females.

The majority of cases which undergo satisfactory surgery in infancy will develop normal speech without needing any specific intervention. **Enderby & Philipp** (1986) estimated that there are 15,000 cleft palate cases in the UK needing help at any one time. In less well developed countries surgery may not always be available or may not be as well advanced, therefore the number of cases with long-term speech problems will be higher. Some babies with severe feeding and respiratory difficulties may not survive. Thus it may be a condition which will present major management problems for clinicians working in the developing world.

Of those infants who have early and successful surgery, around 40 to 50 per cent develop acceptable speech without help (**Van Demark**, 1983). The remainder will have problems for reasons outlined below. In some infants the cleft condition is one of a number of congenital defects, some of which will prevent surgery from being carried out at the optimum time. Children with these conditions may need help over a considerable period of their lives, often into adolescence and even into young adulthood. Even with the provision of good services not all will achieve normal speech.

Types of Cleft and Consequences for Communication

The classification generally used is the one by **Kernahan & Stark** (1958). Clinicians need to be familiar with this as it is frequently used by members of medical and dental teams. Check with others on the classification used. Kernahan and Stark identify three main groups:

1. CLEFTS OF THE PRIMARY PALATE — lip and alveolus;
2. CLEFTS OF THE SECONDARY PALATE — hard and soft palate;
3. CLEFTS OF PRIMARY AND SECONDARY PALATE — both of the above types together.

If we use this classification the groups and the potential consequences for speech are as follows:

Cleft of Lip and Alveolus

This may be unilateral, median or bilateral with the lip and alveolus only involved. The term primary refers to the area anterior to the *incisive foramen* (juncture of pre-maxilla and maxilla), that is the ridge just behind the upper incisors. *Figure 1.1* illustrates a normal palate. Clefts of lip and/or alveolus may indicate that the secondary palate may be at risk, although it appears intact on surface examination.

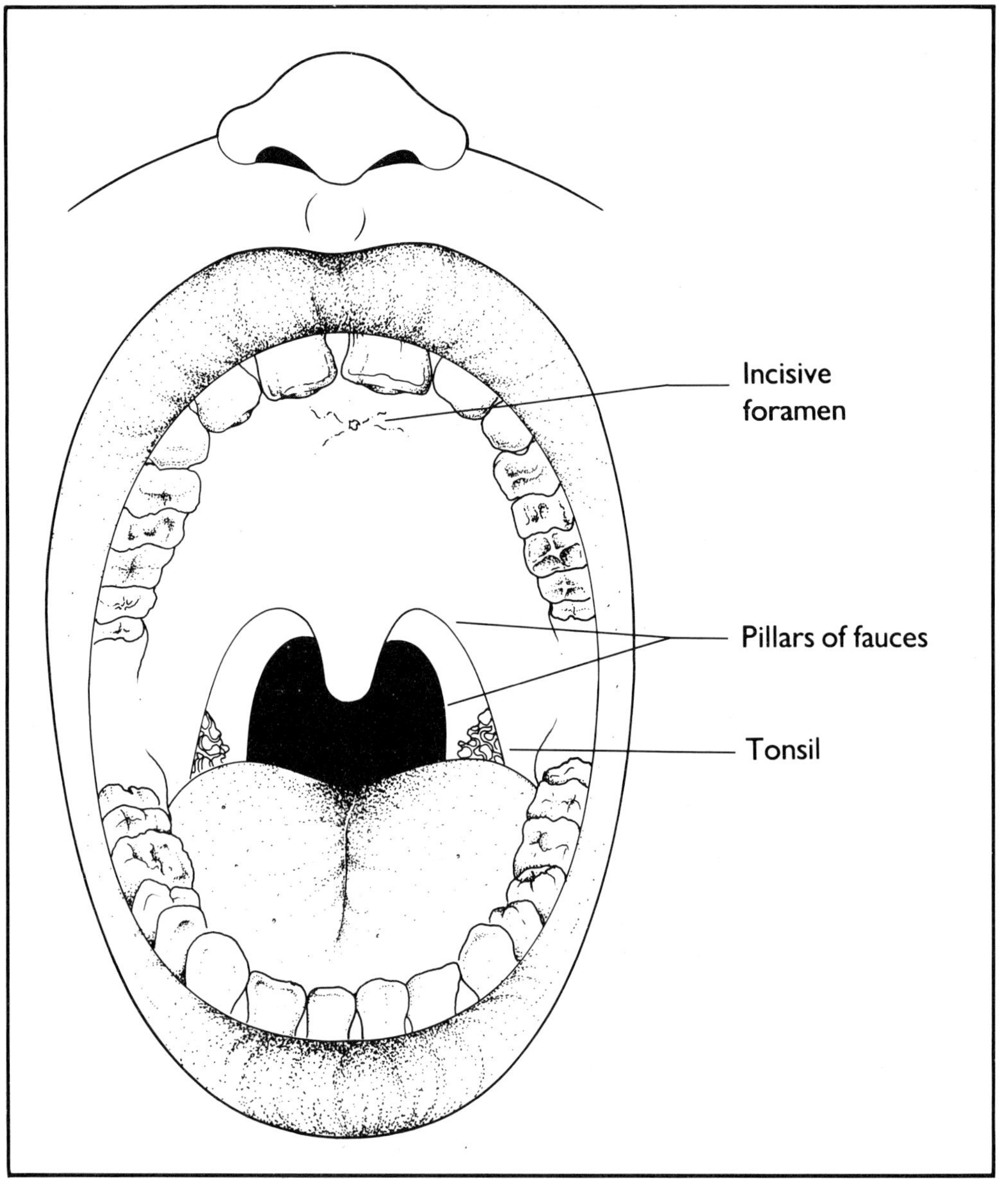

Figure 1.1 **Normal palate**

Potential consequences for speech

Clefts of lip and alveolus only are not likely to be the direct cause of a speech problem, although difficulties might arise because of:

1 Adverse reaction to appearance which could result in poor interpersonal and communication skills.

2 Poor sensory feedback in the area of the cleft of the alveolus, resulting in reduced sensation and imprecise articulation.

3 Wide cleft of the alveolus with consequent dental problems, which may leave a space for the tongue to protrude through, especially in the production of the alveolars /t/d/s/z/.

4 A very tight repaired upper lip which may not be mobile, resulting in restricted movement in speech.

Clefts of the Hard and Soft Palate

The term 'secondary' refers to that part of the palate which lies posterior to the *incisive foramen.* Clefts may be complete, incomplete or sub-mucous. They may therefore involve both the soft and hard palate and range from a bifid uvula (*see Figure 1.2*) to a complete cleft of the hard and soft palate (*see Figure 1.3*).

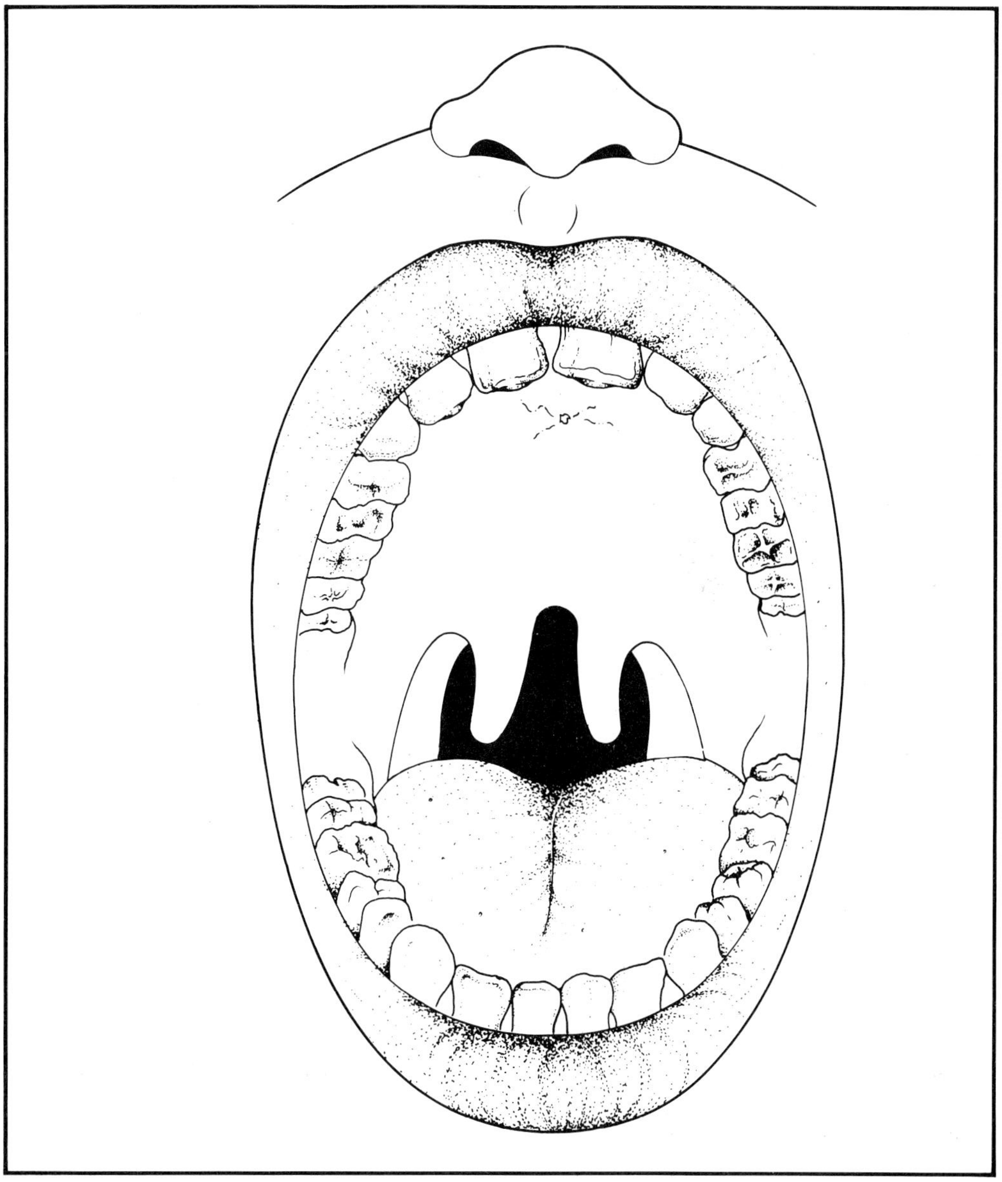

Figure 1.2 **Bifid uvula**

Seemingly insignificant deficiencies in the structure of the uvula are now shown to be of much greater consequence than was previously understood. Diagnostic procedures, such as multiview videofluoroscopy, show that the absence of the musculus uvuli can be associated with velopharyngeal incompetence, when previously the uvula was not considered an essential structure in achieving velopharyngeal closure (**Shprintzen**, 1979).

When children are referred exhibiting resonatory and articulatory problems, there should always be a careful examination for a *sub-mucous cleft* (or other condition affecting the function of the soft palate). Today, in developed countries, a sub-mucous cleft is usually the only cleft which might be missed in the post-natal examination. The condition may not be evident until the onset of speech. There may be defects both in the bones of the hard palate and in the muscles of the soft palate. Although some cases are

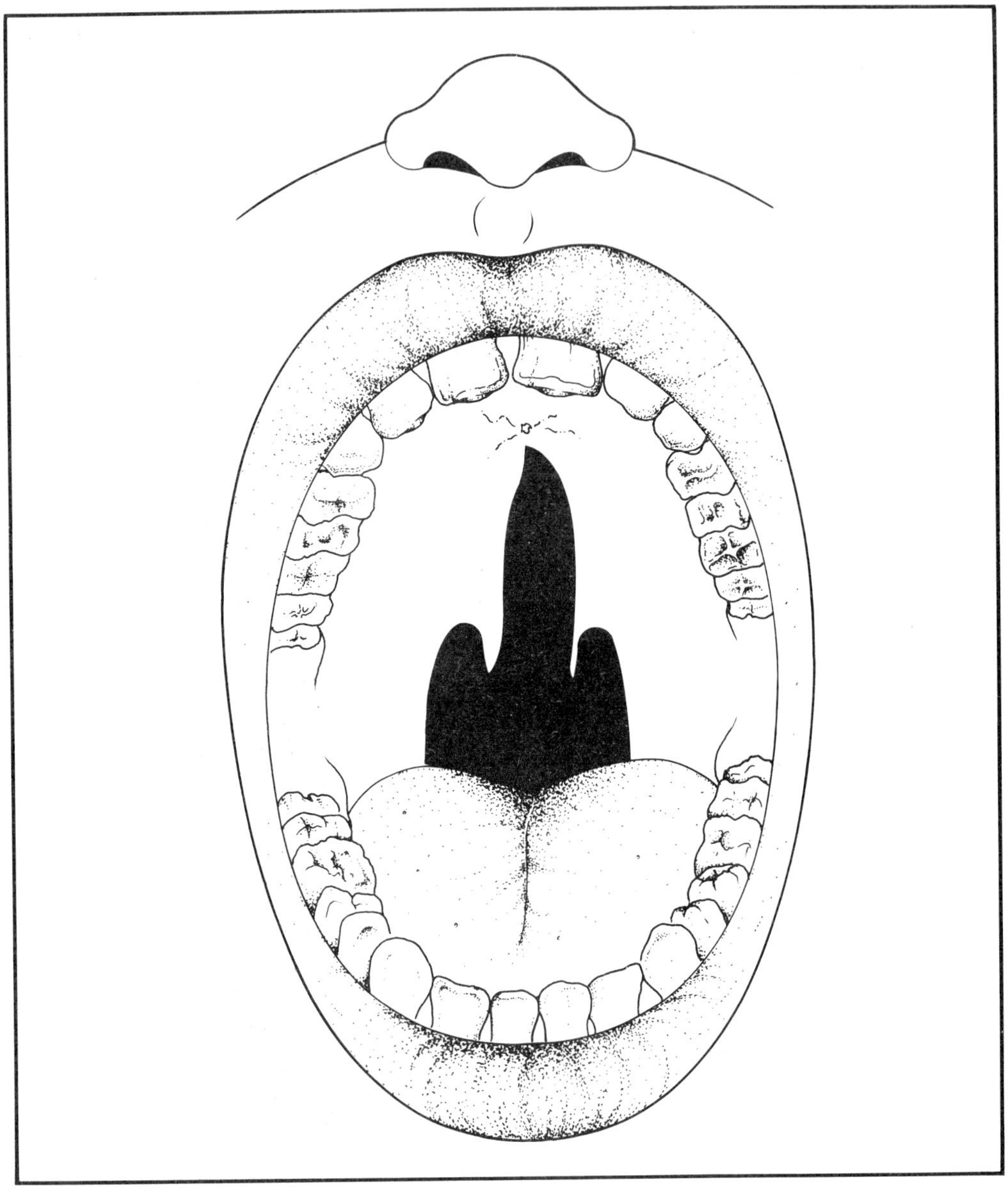

Figure 1.3 **Cleft of soft and hard palate**

reported to be symptom-free, the consequences for speech can be as severe as in an overt cleft.

Potential consequences for speech

1 A bifid uvula may indicate malfunction of the musculus uvuli and may lead to lack of velopharyngeal closure, that is, the soft palate fails to make adequate contact with the pharyngeal wall. This may have severe consequences for speech.

2 In all instances of cleft of the soft palate, velopharyngeal function may be impaired, even after surgery, possibly resulting in a wide range of speech problems at the phonatory, resonatory, articulatory, phonetic and phonological levels. (These will be discussed in *Chapter 2*.)

3 Poor sensory awareness in the area of the hard palate cleft may result in imprecise articulatory placement with phonetic consequences.

4 Some of the clefts of palate only may be extremely wide. Surgery may be difficult and delayed, and may not result in adequate velopharyngeal closure; the effects on speech may be severe, involving all the parameters listed under 2 above.

5 Unrecognised and therefore untreated conditions will lead to the development of deviant speech patterns which become more set as the child

matures. Patterns may be set up which may be difficult to change even when the mechanical cause has been removed.

6 Hearing impairment may also occur which will affect speech and language development.

Complete Clefts

In this category clefts of both the primary and the secondary palates are combined. These may be unilateral, median or bilateral (*see Figure 1.4*). Although the classifications sound straightforward, the actual manifestations may present in many different ways (*see Figure 1.5*). These types of clefts are likely to have wide-ranging physical implications which may have an effect on the development of communication.

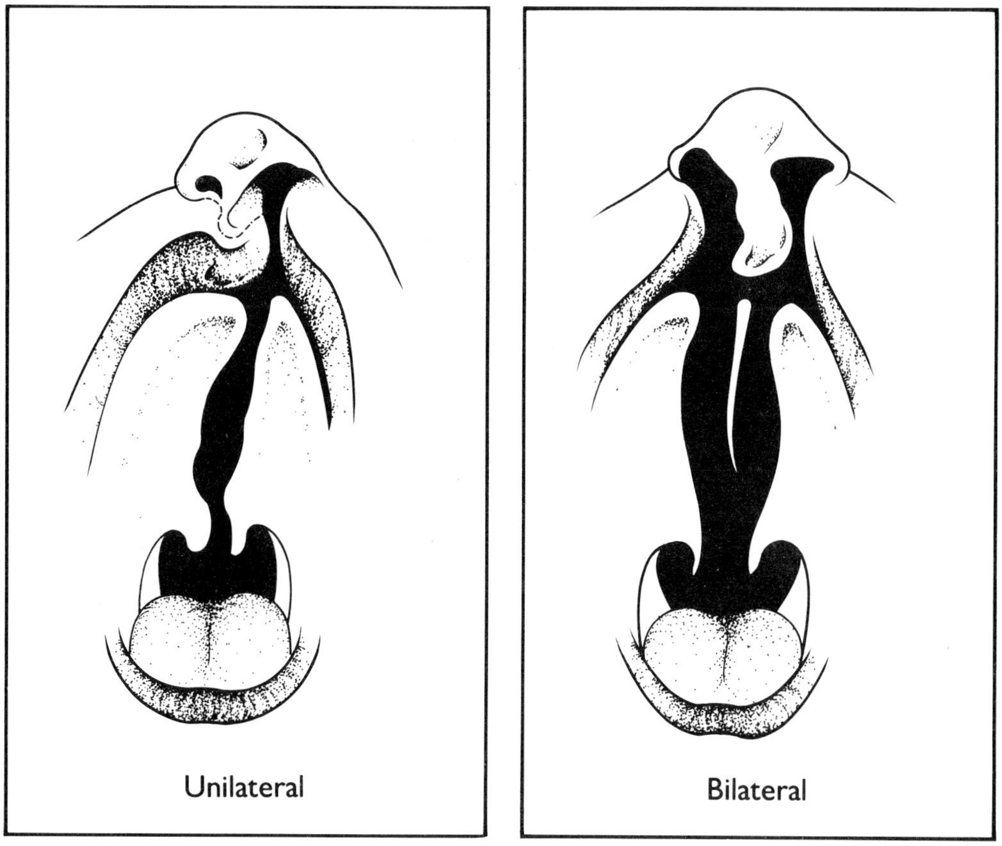

Figure 1.4 **Clefts of primary and secondary palate**

Potential consequences for speech

Although many of these children will, after successful surgery, develop normal communication without any specific help, in some cases there are factors which put normal communication in jeopardy. These include:

1 Adverse reaction to appearance.

2 Low sensory awareness in the hard palate and alveolar ridge, leading to imprecise articulation.

3 Poor velopharyngeal function, post-operatively, leading to phonatory, resonatory, articulatory and phonetic problems.

4 Residual oro-nasal fistula, leading to nasal emission and articulatory problems. (*See page 11.*)

5 Hearing loss, which frequently occurs in clefts involving the soft palate, affecting speech and language development.

6 Speech difficulties secondary to dental malocclusions.

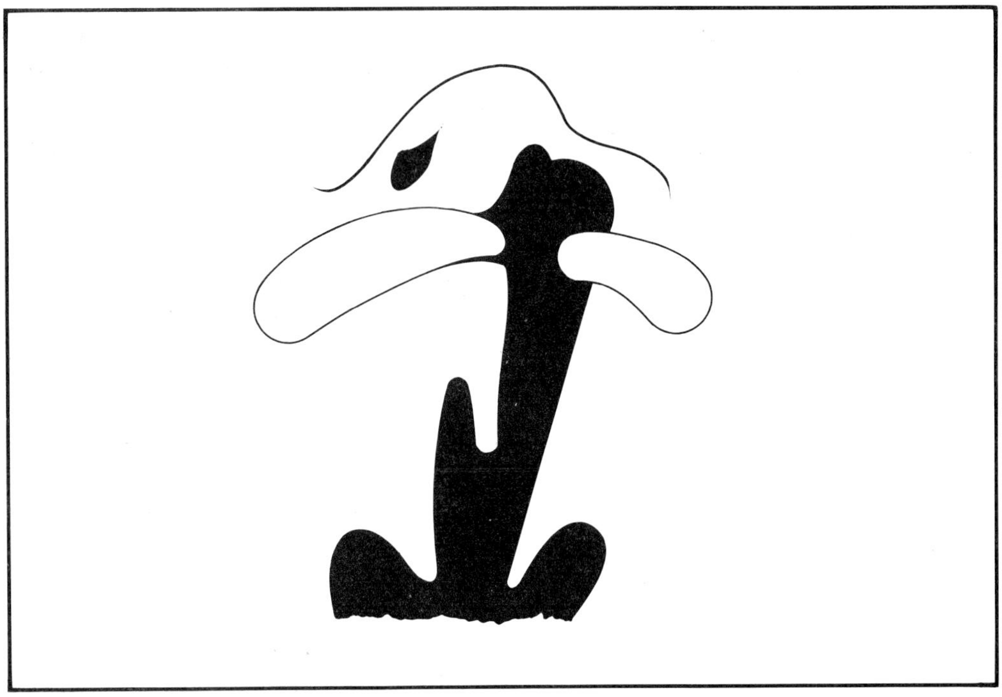

Figure 1.5 ***Example of cleft of primary and secondary palate***

Delayed Surgery

In some of the palatal cleft conditions it may not be possible for the plastic surgeon to undertake operations during infancy. This may be because of other medical problems, such as a heart condition, severe respiratory problems or because the cleft of the soft palate is so extensive that surgery is unlikely to achieve velopharyngeal closure (Pierre Robin syndrome). In some cases there are mechanical limitations, such as restriction on neck extension and mouth opening (Klippel Feil syndrome). Cases of unrepaired cleft palate pose major management and treatment problems for the team.

Congenital Problems Affecting Velopharyngeal Function

There is a further group of cases which must be considered in this section, because, as the speech symptomatology is similar to that found in the cleft palate group, the principles of intervention apply. The major concern with this group is that the condition often goes unrecognised until the maturing infant is well into speech development. These children may show all or some of the following features:

1. Flaccid oro-facial musculature.
2. History of sucking, swallowing, feeding problems.
3. Mild to severe drooling.
4. Weak movement of lips, tongue and palate.
5. Speech problems at the phonatory, resonatory, articulatory and phonetic levels.

These cases are diagnosed as having Congenital Palatopharyngeal Incompetence (CPI). The classification used by **Kaplan** (1975) is useful:

1 *Anatomical disproportion with normal soft palate function.*
The soft palate may be short or the pharynx very deep. Such a condition will require precise diagnosis; in the older child this can be done through

nasendoscopy, if available (*see page 100*), followed by surgery to produce anatomical proportions which can achieve velopharyngeal closure. If advanced diagnostic facilities are not available, the speech manifestations and a period of diagnostic therapy should provide important diagnostic indicators.

2 *Muscle dysfunction with normal proportions.*
This requires precise diagnosis and may require both surgery and other types of intervention, such as Palatal Training Appliance (PTA), and Visual Speech Aid (VSA) (*see Chapter 9*). Cases are likely to have vegetative as well as speech problems. Muscle weakness relates to the malfunction of Cranial Nerves X and XII.

3 *A combination of anatomical disproportion and muscle dysfunction.* Likely to need both surgical and muscle re-education, with severe consequences for both speech and vegetative functions and presenting long-term management problems.

Shprintzen (1979) claims that some of these cases do in fact have a sub-mucous cleft which can be revealed by advanced diagnostic procedures. He therefore questions the above classifications. His view reinforces the need for a thorough anatomical examination.

Speech Problems after Adenoidectomy

After adenoidectomy there is frequently a short period when children present with hypernasality (excess nasal resonance). Occasionally this does not resolve spontaneously. Nasal emission and weakened articulation may also be evident. The history will be of normal speech development, but there may have been feeding problems, including nasal regurgitation. The problems after adenoidectomy may occur because pre-operatively the adenoids helped to occlude the nasopharnyx. Children need diagnosis through nasendoscopy (*see Chapter 4*) and may need surgery to achieve adequate velopharyngeal function. *In cases of cleft palate or CPI, adenoidectomy should only be undertaken with extreme caution.*

Factors Which Have a Major Influence on the Development of Communication

In addition to children experiencing difficulty with speaking as a direct influence of the cleft palate condition, other secondary conditions may occur which further hinder the development of speech. The following are of note:

HEARING IMPAIRMENT

DENTAL MALOCCLUSION

ORO-NASAL FISTULA

Hearing Impairment

The presence of hearing impairment may have serious and wide-ranging effects on the development of speech and language. Furthermore it will be an additional handicap in carrying out remedial procedures. High incidence of middle ear disease and consequent hearing loss have been reported in numerous studies. Otitis media is reported in virtually all cases of unrepaired cleft of palate, by the age of two years (**Paradise**, 1975). This finding will be of major importance in those countries where early surgery may not be available.

Key concepts

- Hearing loss frequently occurs in cases of cleft palate.
- The later the repair, the greater the risk of hearing impairment.
- Hearing loss is usually of a conductive nature and therefore fluctuates.
- Children with CPI, for reasons other than cleft of palate, will also be at risk of hearing impairment.
- Sensorineural loss is occasionally present.
- Where hypertrophied (enlarged) adenoids are implicated as the cause of hearing loss, they should only be removed with extreme caution, as they may be a vital structure in helping to achieve and maintain velopharyngeal closure.

Dental Malocclusion

There is a high incidence of dental malocclusions in individuals with cleft lip and/or palate, because there is a potential for 'gross deformity of the dento-alveolar structures as well as the basal elements of the upper jaw and palate' (**Foster**, 1980). There is some debate as to whether the malocclusion is caused by the original condition or is precipitated or exacerbated by surgical intervention. Individuals with a small maxilla and a comparatively large mandible are not seen as frequently in clinic as formerly; nevertheless some cases still occur. The incidence of malocclusion in unrepaired palatal clefts is being studied in some populations (**Sell & Woodard**, 1987).

The occurrence of a *Class III malocclusion*, in which the mandible is in a forward position to the maxilla, may have a marked effect on phonetic realisation. The mandible is not usually too large but the maxilla is too small, not providing enough space for tongue function in speech. *Figure 1.6* illustrates a Class III malocclusion. As the patient grows the characteristic impaired growth of the maxilla frequently becomes more obvious, resulting in a Class III malocclusion. The following features may be found:

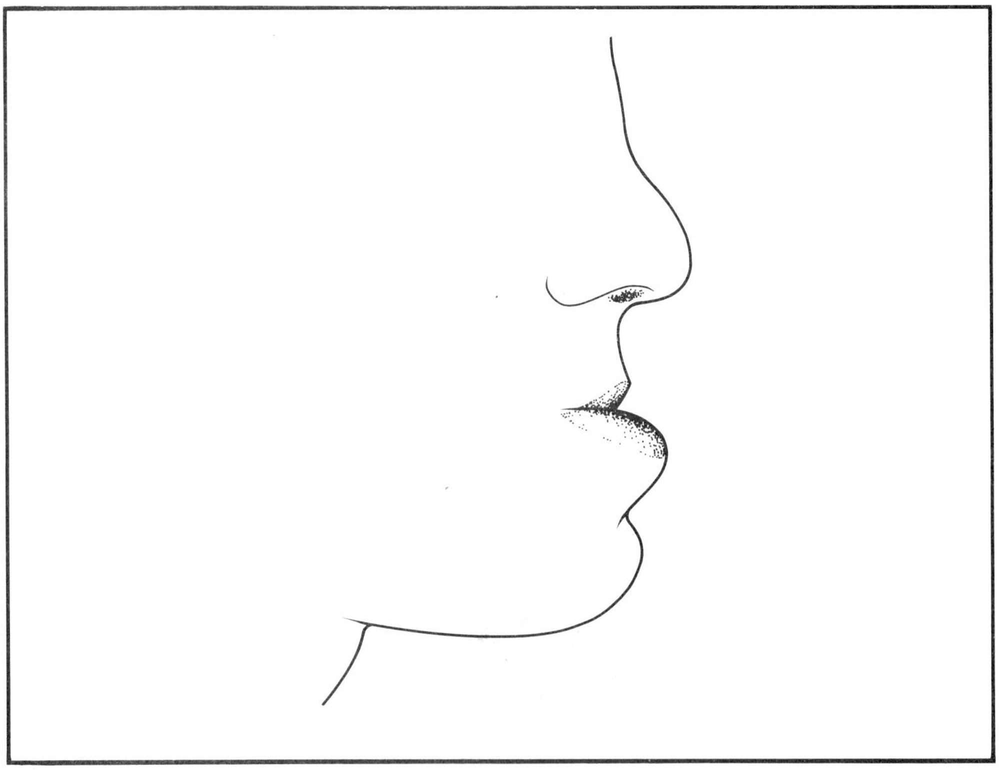

Figure 1.6 ***Profile in Class III malocclusion***

1 Inability/difficulty in achieving a labio-dental position. Maxillary teeth may rest inside the mandible, with lips used as the main articulators, eg. /f/ and /v/ > /Φ/ and /β/; labio-dental is reversed with lower lip to upper teeth: /p̺, b̺, m̺, f̺, v̺/.

2 The tongue cannot be contained within an underdeveloped mandible. The tongue rests in the base of the mandible and the blade of the tongue is used as the main articulator, resulting in palatalisation.

3 Tongue-tip to alveolar ridge contact is difficult to achieve. Precise articulation with central tongue grooving for /s/z/ is not achieved.

4 The sides of the tongue drop down and lateralisation of /s/ and /z/ results.

Other types of malocclusion will be considered in *Chapter 3*, on assessment.

Key concepts

- In older patients (10 upwards) with persisting articulation difficulties, occlusion should be carefully checked.
- Tongue size relates to size of mandible.
- The functional relationship between the maxilla/mandible and tongue should be considered.
- The maxilla needs to provide sufficient space to contain the tongue functioning for speech: width is crucial.
- Class III malocclusion as a possible contributory factor to nasality and/or nasal escape should be considered.

Oro-nasal Fistula

An oro-nasal fistula is an opening in the hard palate which remains after the palate has been repaired; it leads into the nasal passages. It is most frequently situated at the site of the incisive foramen; this is where the surgical flaps meet, and is in fact a breakdown in the original surgical repair. In some cases the repair of the hard palate is deliberately delayed and there is full communication between the oral and nasal cavities. This is illustrated in *Figure 1.7*. In this context, 'fistula' is a misleading term.

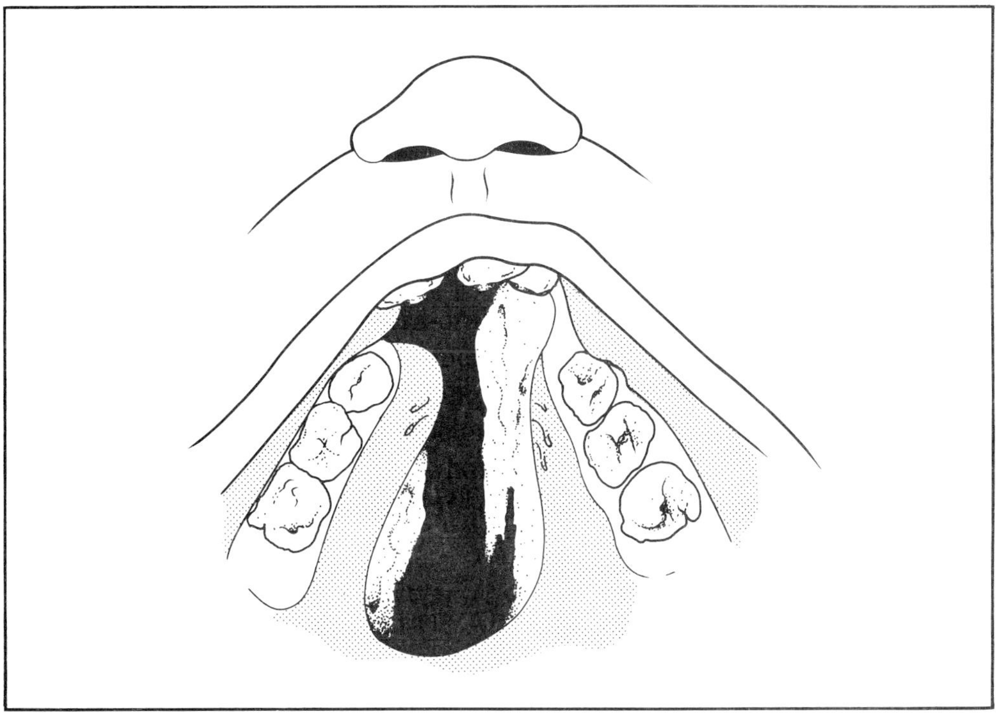

Figure 1.7 **Palatal cleft, where soft palate only has been repaired**

The significance of oro-nasal fistula is not clearly established, although a study of 23 cases by **Stengelhofen & Foster** (1979) did show some evidence of the incidence of both nasal emission and phonetic problems in speech.

Size of fistulae varies considerably and, although there does not appear to be a straightforward relationship between size and the severity of speech problems, there is a clear relationship at the extremes. Where the fistula is difficult to see on surface examination and is only identified by the use of a dental probe, it is unlikely to allow air-flow or liquids into the nose. *Figure 1.8* illustrates a range of fistula shapes and sizes. A large fistula may be the source of air escaping into the nose, although the tongue function may reduce the potential size of the channel. If air is escaping into the nose it is most likely to cause *audible nasal emission* rather than hypernasality. Nasal emission is most likely to occur in association with the production of consonants requiring a high level of intra-oral air pressure, when air will be forced into the nose via the fistula. Surgery to close significant oro-nasal fistulae is now more frequently undertaken. Alternatively, the fistula may be obturated with a dental plate.

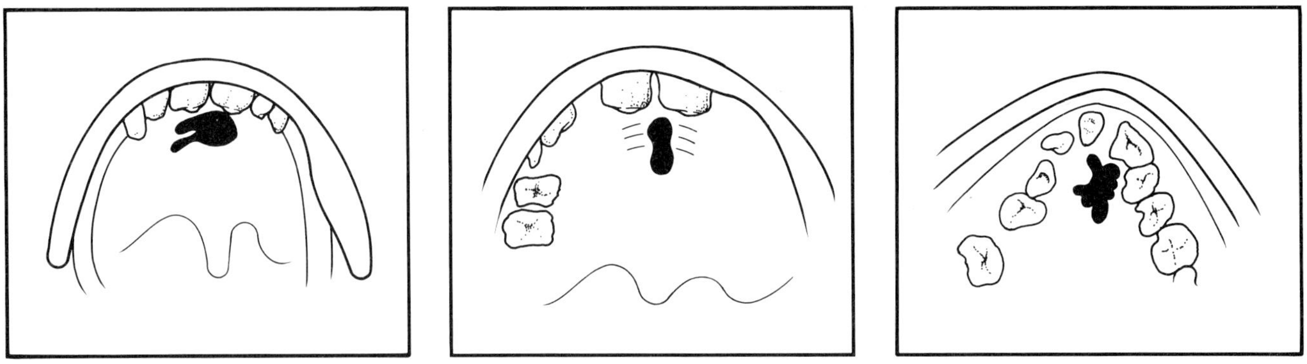

Figure 1.8 **Fistula examples**

Key concepts

- Fistula sizes vary, but the relationship to speech is not clearly established.
- Nasal emission and phonetic problems may result.
- The function of the tongue may be significant in occluding the fistula.
- The maxillary/mandibular relationship may also affect speech.
- It is essential to establish whether air-flow is through the fistula or velopharyngeal mechanism. This can be done through temporary closure of the fistula (*see Chapter 3*).

Is Acceptable Speech Likely to Develop After Surgery?

The majority of children born with cleft lip and palate/cleft palate develop acceptable speech, without help, if successful surgery is carried out in infancy. Why is it, then, that some children who receive surgery at the optimum time have persisting problems? There are several factors which are relevant in developing a prognostic statement. The following questions should be asked:

1. What was the nature and severity of the original condition?
2. When did the surgery take place and what was the experience of the surgeon?
3. Were any particular surgical problems encountered?

4 What were vocalisations/speech like at the time of surgery?

5 What appears to be the status of the vocal tract after surgery? Take particular note of the function of the soft palate.

6 Are there any dental/occlusal problems?

7 What is hearing like?

8 What is the level of sensory awareness?

9 Are there any significant social or psychological factors which will affect the child's progress?

10 What is the child's level of intellectual functioning?

11 What is the emotional adjustment of the family and child to appearance and communication?

12 Are there any other handicapping conditions? What is their nature and severity?

13 Can the necessary services be delivered and what is the efficacy of these services?

14 Are parents likely to be able to co-operate with the services offered?

Finally it should be remembered that the relationship between structure and function is a tenuous one, making speech outcome difficult to predict on the basis of the structure alone. Surprisingly good speech is achieved by some individuals with unrepaired clefts of the palate, in contrast to the poor speech of some individuals who, on examination, appear to have an adequate anatomical structure.

Chapter 2
THE NATURE OF THE SPEECH DIFFICULTIES

Degrees of Nasal Air-flow in Speech / *16*
Resonance / *16*
Phonation / *18*
Articulation / *19*
Phonetic and Phonological Levels / *21*
Intelligibility / *22*
The Incidence of Language Problems / *22*

CHAPTER 2
THE NATURE OF THE SPEECH DIFFICULTIES

In order to remediate the speech problems associated with cleft palate it is necessary to have a thorough understanding of their nature and the mechanisms by which they arise. This chapter is intended as a reminder of the essential concepts as a preparation for practice. Readers are directed to more detailed texts for the theoretical basis.

Degrees of Nasal Air-flow in Speech

There is a range of acceptability in the degree of perceived nasality across accents; for example, American English tends to be more nasalised than British English. It is now understood that the production of oral sounds involves varying degrees of velopharyngeal closure. Vowels are the main carriers of resonatory features and may be nasalised in varying degrees. The nasal consonants /m/n/ŋ//m̥/n̥/ŋ̊/ have full nasal air-flow. All other consonants have very little or no nasal air-flow.

Resonance

Resonance is a perceived feature of speech which is the result of the way the oral and nasal cavities are coupled together. The palate which is cleft or poor in movement has inadequate or no control over this coupling. The three types of resonance are summarised in *Figure 2.1*. A further feature, nasal emission, has been added, because it may be found in cases with velopharyngeal inadequacy, although it is most properly categorised as an articulatory feature.

Nasal emission is different from hypernasality, and should not be confused with it. Emission is the sound of nasal air-flow which sometimes accompanies consonant production. It is most likely to occur in high-pressure consonants. Although the function of the velopharyngeal mechanism is central in the control of resonatory features, there has been a tendency for clinicians to consider palatal function as almost the only factor. **Edwards & Watson** (1980) identified a number of factors which contribute to *hypernasality*:

- Structure of the velopharynx;
- Tongue position;
- Timing and synchrony of movement;
- Hearing and auditory perception;
- Maxillary/mandibular relationship;
- Habit;
- Non-organic.

MECHANISM	SPEECH FEATURES
Normal resonance	
Appropriate well-timed coupling of oro-pharyngeal and nasal cavities.	Acceptable 'normal' speech.
Hypernasality	
Inappropriate/excess coupling of oral and nasal cavities, too much air flows into nose.	Vowels may be hypernasal. Articulation may be normal but may have deviant features of resonance and poor intra-oral air pressure-weakened plosives and fricatives.
Hyponasality	
Insufficient oral/nasal coupling. Not enough air flows into nose because of some form of nasal blockage.	Vowels are hyponasal, as with a cold. Nasals may be affected; eg. /m/>/b/. Articulation becomes generally imprecise because of forward tongue posture from mouth breathing.
Cul-de-sac resonance	
Nasal passage is blocked; when air passes into nose it will be trapped. May be found in cases of velopharyngeal inadequacy where there is also a blocked airway.	Mixture of hyper/hyponasal features. May have both resonatory and articulatory consequences.
Nasal emission	
Air passes into the nose via velopharyngeal sphincter or oro-nasal fistula. Restriction of the nasal passages through tension sets up turbulence and friction becomes audible.	Consonants may be accompanied or replaced by audible nasal emission; nasal grimace may restrict the nares and passages and increase the turbulence.

Figure 2.1 ***Resonatory qualities***

The clinician needs to look at all the potential contributory factors, many of which will be remediable. Surgical intervention may be required, but in some instances surgery to improve the velopharyngeal mechanism may not be possible. It will then be particularly important to attend to the other factors which may be contributing to or maintaining the hypernasality.

Key concepts

- ▶ There are several contributory causes of hypernasality.
- ▶ All causes must be investigated and taken into account in remediation.

The range of resonatory features, together with the mechanisms involved and the resulting speech, should be studied (*see Figure 2.1*). All these features may be found on occasion in cases of cleft palate.

Phonation

Voice problems in children are not always recognised. This is understandable especially where other speech problems are salient and it is difficult to identify all the elements of the problem. In children with cleft palate it is not easy to disentangle phonatory from resonatory qualities. The following phonatory features may be present:

- Weakness (ie reduced loudness/intensity);
- Hoarseness;
- Inappropriate pitch, tendency to higher pitch reported;
- Phonatory breaks;
- Hard glottal attack.

Phonatory problems arise because of the interrelationship between different parts of the vocal tract. Individuals with a problem in one part of the mechanism, eg. the velopharynx, may develop compensatory movements to try to overcome inadequacies. What they are also doing is exacerbating the problem by causing tension which overflows into the whole of the tract and the larynx. *Figure 2.2* summarises the mechanisms which may lead to phonatory changes.

There is laryngoscopic evidence for a high incidence of vocal fold pathology in individuals with cleft palate. It is important for clinicians to be aware of the frequent incidence of phonatory changes.

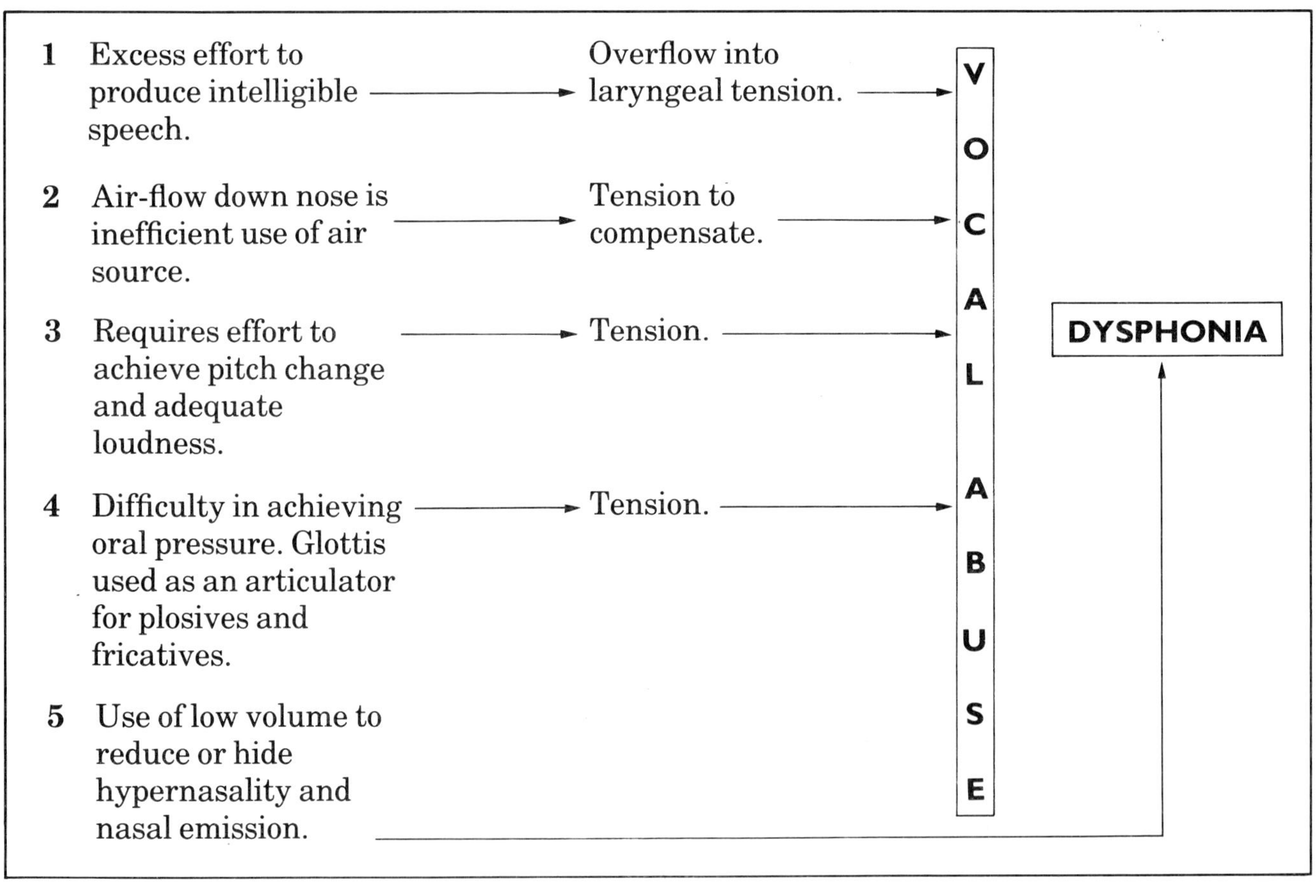

Figure 2.2 ***Abusive mechanisms which may lead to changes in phonation***

Key concepts

- Watch out for voice problems.
- Voice problems may be an important diagnostic feature of inadequate velopharyngeal closure.
- The voice problem needs to be considered as an integral part of the presenting speech problems.
- The dysphonia must be included in the treatment plan.

For further discussion see **Boone** (1982) and **Wilson** (1987).

Articulation

Children with a history of cleft palate have inadequacies in the basic mechanism which is used adaptively to produce speech sounds. The ability to use different articulatory features is necessary in making a distinction between sounds. From an examination of the oral and velopharyngeal structures it is difficult to predict likely speech production. Control has to be achieved over the following articulatory features:

- AIR-STREAM
- MANNER
- VOICING
- PLACE

The potential problems of control of articulatory features are summarised in *Figure 2.3*.

Articulation may be affected by a number of factors, of which the following are of note:

- Velopharyngeal competence;
- Hearing;
- Malocclusion;
- Oro-nasal fistula;
- Sensory awareness;
- Precision of movement;
- Range and strength of movement.

Articulation in cleft palate speakers may show the following features:

1. Improper tongue position during the production of vowels, which may inhibit the achievement of the target positions necessary for the precise articulation of consonants.
2. Poor sensory and spatial awareness in the oral cavity, which reduces the motor control and leads to inaccurate articulation.
3. Tendency for tongue contacts to be retracted.
4. Changes in breath direction.
5. Inadequacy of breath support leading to weakened sound production.
6. Weakened fricatives and plosives.
7. Fricatives and affricates are extremely vulnerable.
8. The presence of audible nasal emission, which may mask a sound which is basically correct in manner and place.
9. Frequent use of glottal stops.
10. Pharyngeal substitutions.
11. The presence of secondary articulations.
12. In Class III malocclusion the dominance of lamino contacts and therefore imprecise articulatory contacts. Lateralisation is frequently found.

13 Relationship between hypernasality and deviant tongue position.

14 Clefts of lip only rarely cause articulation problems. If these are found other causes should also be explored.

15 It is unusual to find difficulties in the production of nasals.

16 Difficulties with glides are occasionally found.

	NORMAL	DIFFICULTY
Air-stream	Control egressive air-stream by velopharyngeal closure, direct air into mouth and create intra-oral air pressure.	Inefficient use of air because of loss into nose. Reduction of air pressure in mouth.
Voicing	Control of +/− voice to produce different consonants.	May not be able to control +/− voicing. Voiceless (fortis) requires more air pressure than voiced (lenis). May not be possible physically. Marked difficulty with fortis.
Manner (*See also Figure 2.4*)	Air modified as it passes up the vocal tract. For oral sounds pressure builds up behind constriction.	In directing air into mouth. Reduced air pressure in mouth creates change of manner.
Place (*Note*: Some places may cause particular difficulties, leading to over- or inappropriate use of some structures.)		
1 ***Glottis***	Only used occasionally as a place of articulation.	Over-use as a place of articulation.
2 ***Labio-dental***	Upper incisors to lower lip.	Class III malocclusion may make contact difficult.
3 ***Alveolar***	A large number of consonants use tongue-tip to alveolar ridge contact.	Poor sensory awareness in alveolar ridge. Tongue bunched in back of mouth and tongue-tip lowered.
4 ***Retroflex***	Ability to lift tongue-tip and curl back. (Retroflex not in English phonetic repertoire.)	Bunching of tongue reduces flexibility of tongue-tip.
5 ***Palatal***	Normally palate surface is intact and smooth.	Hard palate may be unrepaired, scarred or have fistula. Provides a poor contour and insensitive surface.
6 ***Velar and uvular***	Requires intact, mobile soft palate. (Velars only in English.)	Palate may be unrepaired or immobile and/or insensitive. Leads to imprecise contact.
7 ***Pharyngeal***	Not used in English.	As pharynx is below the point of velopharyngeal closure, may be used as a place of constriction for articulation.

Figure 2.3 ***Problems with articulatory features***

A hierarchy of difficulties in the manner of articulation is suggested in *Figure 2.4*.

	MANNER	**EXAMPLE**
MOST DIFFICULT	Plosives	/pbtdkg/
↓	Fricatives	/fvszʃʒΦβ/
	Affricates	/tʃ//dʒ/
	Laterals	/ɬ/
	Rolls/flaps	/ɾ ɽ/
	Glides	/wvlr/
LEAST DIFFICULT	Nasals	/mnŋ/

Figure 2.4 ***Manner of articulation***

Key concepts

- Difficulties with basic articulatory skills produce problems at phonetic and phonological levels.
- Changes in both manner and place need careful analysis.
- Articulatory problems may be very persistent.
- Velopharyngeal competence is central in the ability to achieve articulatory skills.

Phonetic and Phonological Levels

Phonology has been described as a bridge between the phonetic level and other levels of language (**Crystal**, 1980). A difference of meaning is created by using phonetic contrasts. These may be difficult for cases with cleft palate. A reduced sound repertoire (phonetic inventory) places considerable stress on the individual to produce phonological contrasts. Some examples are shown in *Figure 2.5*. Additionally where there is phonetic deviance this may obscure the individual's attempts to signal phonological contrasts. However, if the meaning is not obscured, phonetic differences may not result in phonological problems. In working with cleft palate cases it is necessary to use a fine phonetic transcription, in order to identify any small phonetic differences which may be used to signal meaning (*see Jeremy's case, Chapter 10*). The use of additional symbols, such as is suggested in Phonetic Representation of Disordered Speech, is recommended (**Grunwell**, 1983).

VOICING	
/pɪn/vs/bɪn/	Individual may be unable to make the fortis/lenis contrast.
FINAL CONSONANTS	
bow vs boat /boʊ/vs/boʊt/	Final consonant deletion may be a means of reducing or avoiding nasal emission.
car vs cars /ka:/vs/ka:z/	/z/ may not be in system, or breath may not be sufficient to get to end of word, especially where a high level of intra-oral air pressure is required, as in signalling plurals.

Figure 2.5 ***Phonetic difficulties which may affect the signalling of meaning***

Key concepts

- ▶ Developing phonological processes will be influenced by the physical status and by the normal maturational processes.
- ▶ The signalling of phonological contrasts may be impaired by inability to produce correct phonetic realisations.
- ▶ Linguistic receptive abilities may demonstrate the perceptual awareness of contrasts.

Intelligibility

Intelligibility is a variable feature, sometimes changing from one context or one utterance to another. Listener variables have also been found to have an influence on the judgement of intelligibility. Some sex differences have been noted in individuals with cleft palate, with females tending to be more intelligible than males. In some cases, although a number of speech parameters, including phonetic realisations, are distorted, intelligibility may be preserved. Intelligibility is influenced by a large number of features. It is essential to examine all the contributory features as a basis for treatment. These include:

- ▶ Phonation;
- ▶ Resonance;
- ▶ Articulation;
- ▶ Phonetic features;
- ▶ Phonological ability;
- ▶ Accent;
- ▶ Rate;
- ▶ Prosody;
- ▶ Volume;
- ▶ The number of sounds which are erroneous;
- ▶ The consistency of sound errors;
- ▶ Frequency of occurrence of sounds with errors;
- ▶ Similarity between the errors and the target sound.

The Incidence of Language Problems

Children with cleft lip and/or palate are particularly vulnerable to being delayed or disordered in language development. The following reasons and mechanisms have been put forward:

1 Communication may be adversely affected by a disrupted mother/baby bonding.

2 Hearing impairment is frequently present and will put the development of both speech and language at risk.

3 Frequent periods of hospitalisation, necessary in some cases, may not be conducive to language development.

4 The presence of poor speech in an individual discourages communication with others and the developing child may not be given reinforcement for attempts at talking.

5 Adults may not understand the child and misconstrue intended meaning, which will cause confusion. There may be limited opportunity for modelling and expanding the child's unintelligible utterances.

6 Children with poor speech may lack confidence and be unwilling to use language.

7 The natural protectiveness of some parents may discourage children from expressing themselves.

8 Some individuals with inadequate or deviant speech use reduced word and sentence length and simplified sentence structures in an attempt to preserve intelligibility.

Intellectual impairment is recognised as a cause of delayed language development, but it could also be a factor in relation to a child's ability to adapt to an inadequate mechanism. However it should be noted that the suggestion that intellectual impairment has a high incidence in individuals with cleft palate is not supported by recent research evidence (**Heinmann-de Boer**, 1985).

Although the incidence of language delay in these children is of major importance, it is an area which will not be addressed further in this book, because there is an extensive literature on the description, identification and treatment of language problems in children. The principles discussed in the literature are equally applicable to the assessment and remediation of language in children who have cleft lip and/or palate (see **Cooke & Williams**, *Working with Children's Language*, 1985, in this series).

CHAPTER 3
ASSESSMENT OF THE SPEECH MECHANISM

The Need for a Physical Examination /*26*
Causal Relationships /*27*
General Observations of the Individual /*27*
What to Look for in the Oro-facial Examination /*27*
The Lips /*27*
The Mouth Opening /*29*
The Tongue /*29*
The Nose /*30*
Adenoidal Growth /*30*
Dentition and Occlusion /*30*
The Hard Palate /*31*
The Soft Palate /*32*
The Examination of the Swallowing Pattern /*34*
Diadochokinetic Rates (DDK) /*34*
Sensitivity of the Oral Structures /*35*
The Assessment of Speech /*35*
Principles for the Collection, Analysis and Evaluation of Speech Data /*36*
Phonetic Transcription /*37*
Phonetic Analysis /*37*
Phonological Analysis /*37*
Additional Factors Related to Speech Assessment /*38*
Hearing and Auditory Perceptual Skills /*38*

CHAPTER 3
ASSESSMENT OF THE SPEECH MECHANISM

The Need for a Physical Examination

The relationship between structure and function is a tenuous one. However, as the tract from the larynx to the lips is used adaptively to produce speech sounds, there is a presumption that the actual structure impinges in some degree on the ability of the individual to produce acceptable speech. There are of course many other factors which influence the individual's ability to produce speech.

Where an individual presents with a speech problem, an oro-facial examination should be routinely carried out. If children are difficult to understand, an examination of the speech mechanism should always be undertaken, to ascertain that anatomical factors are not present which may be detrimental to speech development. It is unwise to presume that the presenting speech problem is at the phonological level: *if in doubt carry out an examination of the peripheral speech mechanism.*

Speech description and evaluation needs to be approached from a number of different angles, which are illustrated in *Figure 3.1*. The examina-

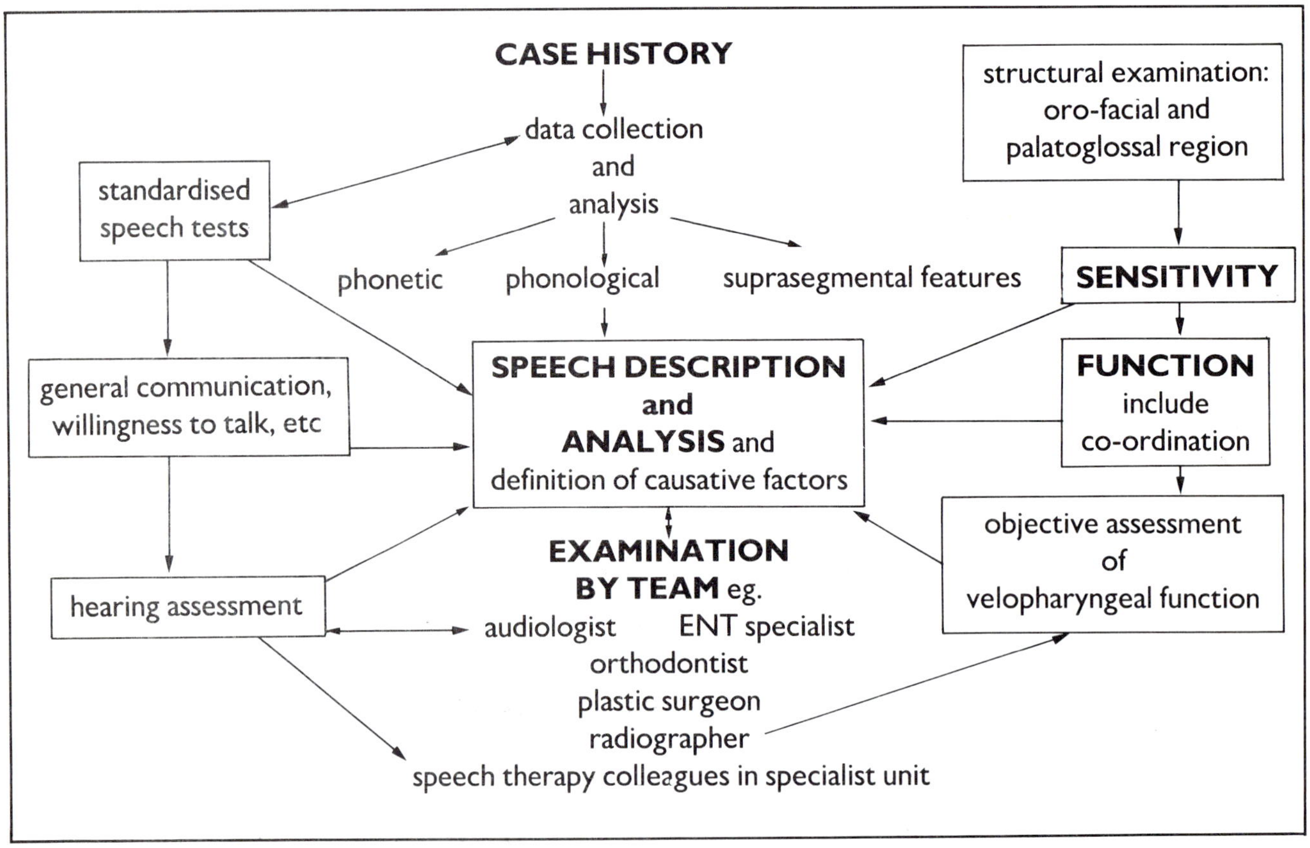

Figure 3.1 ***Ways of evaluating speech***

tion of the peripheral speech mechanism is one angle, but an essential one in the precise identification of the nature and cause of the speech problem.

Physical examination in the individual with a cleft lip and/or palate needs to be backed up by a team which will help in identifying causative and contributory factors (*see Chapter 4*). The clinician's main job is to identify the need for further examinations. The precise description of the nature of the problem is an essential first step in deciding a management plan. Attention should be given to the following:

- The patient as a whole;
- The maxillo-facial region;
- The velopharyngeal region;
- The larynx.

If dysphonia is identified, referral to the ear, nose and throat (ENT) specialist should be arranged for examination of the status of the larynx.

Causal Relationships

Before starting the physical examination of the patient it should be remembered that *the coexistence of factors does not mean that they are necessarily in a causal relationship*. For example, if a child is found to have a tongue tie this may not mean that it is the cause of the speech problem which is also present. Furthermore some speakers are capable of surmounting seemingly major physical anomalies of the oro-facial region, while others who have minimal anatomical differences exhibit marked dysfunction. The range of speech standards in adults with unrepaired cleft palate demonstrates this, some individuals achieving a remarkable standard of intelligible speech.

It is not wise to set out with any preconceived ideas; examination of the structure and speech description should be carried out as separate pieces of investigation, then the possible links between structure and function may be considered. **Huskie** (1989) provides a useful checklist for the examination of the oro-facial and palato-pharyngeal regions, which should be referred to. Valuable checklists and discussions can be found in **Peterson *et al*** (1981); **Ruscello *et al*** (1982) and **Weiss *et al*** (1980). It is helpful to see the examination findings at a glance; a proforma for this purpose is provided in *Appendix I*.

General Observations of the Individual

Useful observations of the patient, especially the young child, can begin in the waiting area, while talking to the parents or during play. Before attempting to carry out an intra-oral examination there is much which can be observed informally, with the more invasive parts of the examination left until last, with all ages. With young children, time will need to be spent in gaining the child's trust. With older children, adult patients and parents, time should be spent explaining what you are going to do and the purpose of the examination. *Figure 3.2* indicates what may be observed informally.

What to Look for in the Oro-facial Examination

The Lips

Lip abnormalities can be both anatomical and physiological. At rest the lips should provide an anterior oral seal (lip competence). In normal function lips

THE FOLLOWING OBSERVATIONS CAN BE MADE WITHOUT REQUIRING THE CO-OPERATION OF THE PATIENT.	
1	General head and body posture.
2	General co-ordination.
3	Facial appearance — muscle tone, flaccidity, asymmetry etc.
4	Lip posture, presence of lip scars, drooling.
5	Physical abnormalities in the head and neck region, which may be indicative of intra-oral differences, including the possible presence of a syndrome.
6	When patient speaks, the presence of a nasal grimace may be observed. Size and shape of nose.
7	Signs of hearing impairment.

Figure 3.2 ***Informal observations***

only contract very slightly during chewing and swallowing. In aberrant function the lower lip, especially the mentalis muscle, contracts vigorously during swallowing, while the upper lip is passive, the anterior oral seal is maintained by the activity of the mentalis or by the lower lip coming into contact with the upper incisors. Sometimes the tongue is held between the incisors to form a seal. *Figure 3.3* summarises lip abnormalities. Starred (☆) items are of particular significance in cleft lip, while abnormalities of function may be found in individuals with velopharyngeal incompetence (VPI) of neurological origin.

The structure of the lips will have been observed informally. The

STRUCTURE	
1	☆ Under-development of lips.
2	☆ Disease, trauma; eg. absence of tissue following surgery for lip pits.
3	☆ Excessive fullness of lower lip; imbalance of appearance.
4	Lack of fullness of upper lip, especially post-surgery in repaired cleft lip.
5	Problems with closure because of proclined incisors, trapped lip preventing bilabial lip seal.
FUNCTION	
1	☆ Immobility, especially of a tight scarred upper lip.
2	Weak function in speech.
3	Excessive function in vegetative activities.
4	Asymmetry of muscle contraction.
5	Open lip posture.

Figure 3.3 ***Lip abnormalities***

individual should be asked to drink and eat (eg. crisps), to permit observation of lip activity in swallowing and chewing. The function of lips and tongue are closely related. Any excess movement of lips in vegetative function should alert the clinician to possible malfunction of the tongue (see below). The balance of lips, tongue and cheek activity is especially important during the years of development of the face, having a major influence on moulding and holding in balance the structures of the upper and lower jaws. Once established, aberrant lip posture tends to be resistant to change.

The Mouth Opening

Where abnormalities of mouth opening are found, they will frequently coexist with other abnormalities, perhaps as one of the features of a syndrome. Cleft lip and/or palate may also be found. The following variations in mouth opening may be found:

Microstomia, or small mouth opening. Often found in association with a small tongue and mandible. Speech may be inhibited, while reduction in mouth opening leads to increased hypernasality.

Macrostomia results from incomplete fusion of the maxillary and mandibular processes. Speech problems are not associated with macrostomia, although they may be present as a result of cleft palate and/or dental malocclusion, frequently found in association with macrostomia.

In Pierre Robin syndrome the mouth opening is frequently small, in Treacher Collins large, and in Klippel Feil syndrome there tends to be an asymmetrical mouth opening which is restricted because of lack of neck extension. All three conditions may have cleft palate. The associated abnormalities of mouth opening may be an additional hazard to speech development.

The Tongue

Ankyloglossia, or tongue tie, is a handicap if the shortness of the lingual frenum restricts the movement of tongue-tip. It is not easy to assess this in infants. Tongue-tip movement is required for feeding, oral hygiene and speech. Tongue tie has been reported in some cases of Pierre Robin syndrome.

If necessary, surgery for a tongue tie should be undertaken before school age. It is not as simple a procedure as was previously thought, requiring muscle resection of the frenum after freeing of the muscle attachment. Inappropriate surgery can lead to ulceration and excess mobility.

It is essential to examine the size of the tongue as it relates to the mandible and the function as it relates to the maxilla. In some conditions, eg. Down's syndrome the tongue tends to be large. *Figure 3.4* lists points to consider in the assessment of tongue size.

While they are developing speech, children may be able to make major adjustments to anatomical deficiencies of the tongue, providing they have the intellectual ability and are not handicapped by other physical limitations.

Tongue function

Neurological involvement, as found in some conditions which affect the function of the velopharynx, may also involve weak tongue movement.

1	Crenation/notching of the edges of the tongue may indicate large size, rather than being a feature of the function.
2	Large tongue tends to be poorly co-ordinated.
3	If the maxilla is comparatively small there may not be enough space for tongue in speech.
4	The activity of the tongue will be obvious in swallowing and chewing.
5	Articulation will be imprecise, with a tendency to use lamino contacts.
6	Tongue will take up an interdental resting position.

Figure 3.4 ***Assessment of tongue size***

The Nose

The surface structure of the nose can easily be evaluated through informal observation of the patient. It may be obvious that the airway is inadequate because of the size and shape of the nose and because mouth breathing is evident. It is important first to see if the child can provide a clear airway. Many young children do not find it easy to learn to blow their nose. Learning to do this must be a first step to assessing the adequacy of the airway (*page 76*). Features such as a saddle or crooked nose or a collapsed nostril on the side of the cleft will be noted. Blockage of the airway will lead first to mouth breathing, which will in turn lead to a number of other features, for example:

- The maxillary arch narrows, the face also becoming elongated and narrow;
- The mandible drops to an open position;
- Tongue drops to a lowered posture;
- Nostrils become narrowed, leading to an even poorer airway;
- Resonance lacks nasality;
- Articulation becomes imprecise, the tongue blade being used for articulation;
- Hearing loss may lead to further speech difficulties.

Adenoidal Growth

The most common cause of nasal blockage is adenoidal growth. Adenoids usually atrophy, becoming extinct or fibrosclerotic by about 16 years of age, although this does not always happen and infected lymphoid tissue can become hypertrophic and serve as a focus of infection, blocking the nasal airway and leading to hearing loss. Nasal blockage in individuals with a cleft palate, even in the presence of velopharyngeal incompetence, may occur and lead to 'cul-de-sac' resonance, as well as causing conductive hearing loss. The other speech characteristics resulting from nasal blockage, described above, may also be present. Referral should be made to the ENT specialist for investigation of the status of the adenoids.

Dentition and Occlusion

It is necessary to examine the maxilla–mandible relationship at rest, during speech and in swallowing. The patient should be asked to bite down on the back teeth and spread the lips to provide a view. This posture usually produces a pattern of closure characteristic for the individual. Care should be taken that the mandible has not been postured forward to bring the upper and lower incisors together. In the 'normal' bite, in fully-grown individuals, the maxilla is slightly greater in diameter than the mandible, therefore the upper arch teeth overlap the mandibular teeth. Variations may occur:

1 The mandibular base is set back in comparison to the maxilla — *Class II malocclusion (distocclusion)*.
2 There is excessive protrusion of the mandible, so that the lower arch teeth overlap the upper arch — *Class III malocclusion (mesiocclusion)*.
3 *Open bite*, where there is lack of contact between the upper and lower anterior teeth when the back teeth are in occlusion.

Malocclusions in individuals with cleft lip and/or palate are frequently a primary cause of articulatory and phonetic problems (*see Figure 3.5*).

TYPE	TONGUE POSTURES	SPEECH
Class II	forward tongue position associated with tooth position	fronted or dentalised consonants
Class III	tongue-tip remains lowered	labio-dental difficulty; blade used as main articulator
Anterior open bite	with tongue thrust forward in speech	fronted articulation
Note: PRDS use + = advanced, ⁀ = dental/labio-dental, ‿ = reverse labio-dental.		

Figure 3.5 **Speech in malocclusion**

The presence of irregular *dentition* is not likely to cause speech difficulties; however a large space in the dentition, such as may be found at the site of a repaired or unrepaired cleft of the alveolus, may provide a space for the tongue to move into when the target placement is alveolar. Alveolar sounds will then be fronted.

Clinicians should note the presence of teeth in unusual places, for example in the alveolus or in the surface of the hard palate. These may be supernumerary or may be malpositioned teeth. Growth of a tooth in a site used for articulatory placement, such as the alveolar ridge, may interfere with the precise placement necessary for clear articulation.

Neither congenitally missing teeth (in edentulous patients) nor complete absence of teeth (anodontia) are likely to be the prime cause of a speech difficulty. Where the speech clinician identifies dental or occlusal problems, referral should be made to the dental specialist if liaison with a team orthodontist has not already been established (*see Chapter 4*).

The Hard Palate

Examination of the alveolar ridge can be undertaken alongside that of the dentition. The alveolar ridge needs special attention because it is the place of articulation for several consonants. Where scarring is present, sensitivity should be checked.

The incisive foramen is a vulnerable point and may be the site of an oro-nasal fistula (*see Chapter 1*). The maxillary arch and hard palate should be assessed for contour and width. The often cited high palatal vault is not a problem with regard to speech, but the presence of the narrowed maxillary arch which accompanies it provides insufficient space for the tongue to carry out articulatory movements. *Figure 3.6* gives pointers to the hard palate examination. A good view of the hard palate can best be obtained with a mouth examination mirror.

Where an oro-nasal fistula is present, the plastic surgeon and/or orthodontist should be consulted with regard to the long-term management — surgery or dental plate to obturate the fistula.

1	Note intactness and sensitivity of alveolar ridge.
2	Contour and width of palatal vault.
3	Scarring.
4	Presence of oro-nasal fistula.
5	Colour — blueish central zone (zona pallucida) may indicate the presence of a sub-mucous cleft.
6	Presence of misplaced or supernumerary teeth.

Figure 3.6 **Hard palate examination**

The Soft Palate

It is not easy to get a view of the soft palate without getting the patient to open the mouth wide. This usually results in the tongue being raised and the view of the palate being obstructed. When the head is tipped back, normal muscle action may become distorted. Nevertheless it is essential that an examination of the soft palate is attempted. The evaluation of *length* and *mobility* is of prime importance. A wide variation within the normal can be observed in palate length, pharyngeal depth and mobility of the structures.

The soft palate and the uvula should be observed first of all at rest, noting the length and the presence of any scarring. The presence of a bifid uvula should be noted. This may be an indicator of the presence of a sub-mucous cleft, or some other inadequacy of the velopharyngeal structures. Asymmetry of the soft palate at rest should be noted, as this may be an indicator of muscle weakness.

Examination of soft palate movement should be attempted on vocalisation. A tongue spatula or finger may be used to depress the tongue. *The tongue should not be protruded during the examination, since this position will cause movement of the palato-glossal muscle and restrict the elevation of the soft palate during phonation.* Weakness, asymmetry and lack of movement should be recorded. Diadochokinetic rates should be taken. Diadochokinesis is the ability to carry out repeated movements. It is used in a range of neurological examinations and has been adapted for use with the speech mechanism.

Notching or weakness in the uvula muscle can lead to air leak into the nose. The uvula should therefore be examined carefully for notching, bifurcation, size and movement. Surface observation is of limited diagnostic value and should not be used alone as a basis for deciding about the adequacy of the velopharyngeal mechanism. The speech clinician's examination is a screening procedure which attempts to identify features which require further objective investigations.

The gag reflex should be elicited by placing pressure on the back of the tongue or touching the soft palate. Although some normal speakers have depressed gag reflex, lack of sensitivity and the absence of reflex has been noted in a number of individuals with cleft palate.

Movement of the pillars of fauces should be observed during phonation, as the muscles forming the pillars contribute to velopharyngeal closure (*see Figure 1.1*). The presence of tonsils will be apparent during this part of the examination. Tonsils are located between the anterior and posterior pillars of fauces. In some instances they become so enlarged (hypertrophied) that they almost come into contact in the midline. This may have consequences for soft palate function (*see Figure 3.7*).

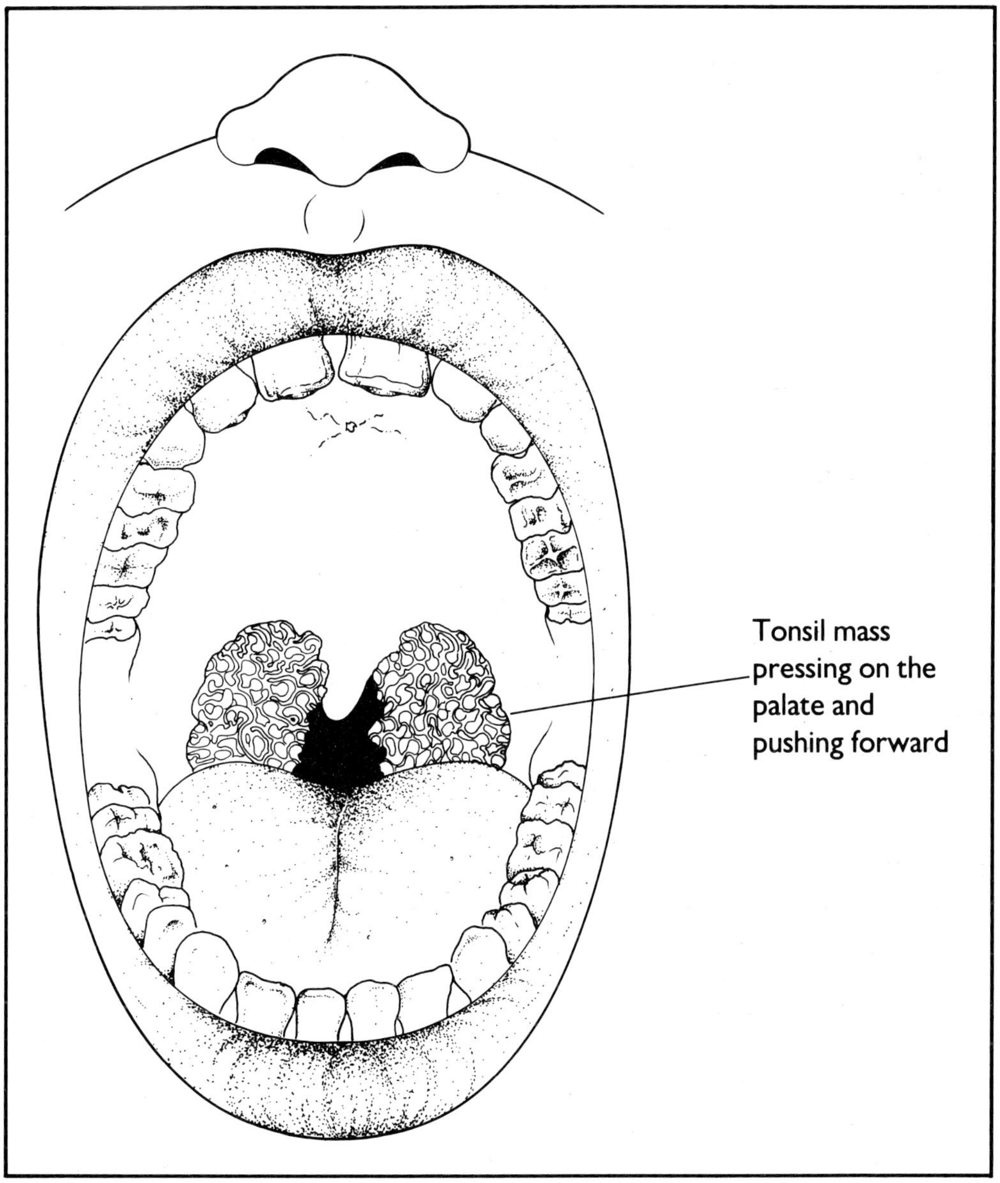

Figure 3.7 **Large tonsils**

Pointers to the examination of the soft palate, uvula and pharynx are included in *Figure 3.8*. The function of the velopharyngeal mechanism is central in the acquisition and maintenance of normal speech. It is imperative that any signs of possible inadequacy should be thoroughly investigated by the specialist team.

STRUCTURE	
1	Length of soft palate.
2	Bifid or absence of uvula.
3	Capacious nasopharynx.
4	Presence of tonsils.
5	Notice scarring of palate and uvula.
FUNCTION	
1	Mobility of the soft palate, uvula and pharyngeal walls.
2	Movement noticed on phonation, but asymmetrical.
3	Examine sensitivity in the immobile palate.
4	Check gag reflex.

Figure 3.8 ***Examination of the soft palate, uvula and pharynx***

The Examination of the Swallowing Pattern

Swallowing is a function which involves a number of the structures mentioned above. Malfunction of the structures may be indicated in aberrant swallowing patterns. The patient should be observed chewing and swallowing. Excessive activity of the lips should be noted. Ask the patient to take a small amount of water into the mouth and hold it until told to swallow. While swallowing is in progress the clinician should open the patient's lips, by depressing the lower lip with the thumbs to move upper and lower lips apart. In the aberrant swallow the lips may be resistant, because of the excess muscle activity. Once the lips are apart the tongue will be exposed if it is protruding through the incisors. The patient should be asked to swallow with water several times. Individuals with a tongue thrust swallow will find it almost impossible to swallow with open lips.

In addition to the structural examination of the speech mechanism, the individual's ability in speech will provide some insight into the features of (a) rate and range of movements; (b) precision of movements; and (c) co-ordination of movements. Not many tests have been standardised for the assessment of these abilities, apart from those for diadochokinetic rates.

Diadochokinetic Rates (DDK)

If the clinician observes aberrant vegetative functions and slow, laboured or indistinct speech, then the basic motor control should be assessed further. DDK rates should be assessed routinely in cases of cleft palate. The relationship between DDK rates and speech is not yet clearly established. It is, however, a measure which many clinicians find valuable. In the UK the norms developed by **Canning & Rose** (1974) are used. Norms have also been supplied by **Fletcher** (1978). The procedure is summarised in *Figure 3.9*.

Take note of any unusual features, such as:

1 Predominance of lingual convexity as the permanent posture from which articulatory placements are made.

2 Tendency to front the tongue and use lamino contacts.

3 Obvious mandibular movements which cannot be suppressed during lingual DDK performance, the mandible carrying the tongue to the articulatory placement.

4 Depression of the lingual tip during /t/d/n/.

5 Inconsistency of movements; imprecise lingual movements, tongue-tip deviations and rotations.

6 Overflow movements.

EQUIPMENT			
Stopwatch Tape recorder			
METHOD			
1	Make sure that the subject understands the nature of the repetition task, and what is required.		
2	For lips: For tongue: For velum:	/pʌ/ /pʌ/ /pʌ/ ten times /tʌ/ /tʌ/ /tʌ/ ten times /kʌ/ /kʌ/ /kʌ/ ten times	speed measured in seconds for ten repetitions on one breath.
3	Repetition of consonant/vowel sequence: /pʌ/ /tʌ/ /kʌ/ speed measured in seconds for ten repetitions.		
For details and norms, see **Canning & Rose** (1974). **Fletcher** (1972) uses a wider range of consonants, including /f/ and /l/.			

Figure 3.9 ***Assessment of DDK rates***

Sensitivity of the Oral Structures

For the production of clear speech it is necessary for the movable articulators to make precise contacts with other organs. Precise contacts depend not only on movement but also on the sensitivity of the organs involved. There is an established relationship between sensitivity and mobility. The tongue-tip should be the most highly sensitive and mobile structure in the mouth. As the tongue needs to contact specific points on the palate it is also necessary for the palate to be sensitive. The alveolar ridge is the most sensitive region, thus tongue-tip and alveolar ridge are key points for articulation. Sensitivity may be assessed by light touching with cotton wool.

A number of complex procedures have been developed, but are not recommended for routine use because the relationship between the findings and speech production is not yet clearly established. Tests for oral form discrimination are the most frequently used, although their validity is not yet fully established.

The Assessment of Speech

In the collection and analysis of speech data the same principles apply to cases with cleft palate as with other disorders. Pointers to the assessment of speech follow. When assessment is completed, the findings should be considered alongside the findings of the examination of the speech mechanism.

Principles for the Collection, Analysis and Evaluation of Speech Data

1 Always use a high-quality tape recorder.

2 Collect a range of data with samples from free speech and standardised procedures.

3 Select procedures appropriate to the age of the individual.

4 Involve the parents as much as possible in the collection of speech data of children.

5 Suggested procedures for articulation:

- ▶ Flash cards;
- ▶ Templin–Darley Test of Articulation (**Templin & Darley**, 1969);
- ▶ Goldman–Fristoe Test of Articulation (**Goldman & Fristoe**, 1972);
- ▶ Edinburgh Articulation Test (EAT, **Anthony *et al***, 1971).

Tests must be used which include samples of a number of pressure consonants (/p/b/t/d/s/z/ʃ/ʒ/). The Templin–Darley test is particularly useful for this. The use of the qualitative analysis in the EAT is of particular importance; children with speech problems secondary to cleft palate may show a number of realisations in the deviant column.

6 With older children and adults reading aloud should be recorded. This provides data for analysis as well as a base-line record for comparison. **Fletcher**'s (1972) and **Boone**'s (1982) reading passages can be used.

7 To collect a brief sample, name, counting to ten, days of the week and months of the year may be collected. This provides a useful base-line and indicates areas for further data collection.

8 From the data collected make judgements of the following:

- ▶ Intelligibility;
- ▶ Phonation;
- ▶ Resonance and nasal emission;
- ▶ Articulatory features.

9 Work out the phonetic inventory from data gathered.

10 Use repetition to give more data in uncertain areas.

11 Carry out a stimulability test. Note that individuals who are aware of their poor speech may change the realisation of a consonant at each successive attempt.

12 Note the following in connected speech:

- ▶ Rate;
- ▶ Volume;
- ▶ Degree of mouth opening;
- ▶ The presence of a nasal grimace;
- ▶ Resonance;
- ▶ Phonation.

Clinicians are sometimes reluctant to ask individuals to do further tasks where they think production may be suspect. It is essential that sufficient data are collected to reveal the patient's difficulties as well as to indicate the potential for improvement.

Phonetic Transcription

Individuals with speech problems from cleft palate will make demands on the clinician's phonetic skills. It should always be remembered that conventional transcription is based on the production of speech with a 'normal structure' and phonetic representations may not fully cover the inventory of individual cases. Time should not be lost in trying to write a particular symbol, which can always be checked later; instead note should be made of relevant features, including place, manner and voicing. In addition to audio-recording, as much as possible should be transcribed at the time. This should include ratings to indicate the severity of resonatory features, as well as features of velarisation, pharyngealisation, lateralisation, nasal emission and snort, and nasal grimace.

Use of the Phonetic Representation of Disordered Speech is recommended (**Grunwell**, 1983) to provide additional symbols to be used in the transcription. The following symbols may be found to be particularly useful:

- Labio-dentals /p̪/ /b̪/ /m̪/;
- Reverse labio-dentals /p̺/ /b̺/ /m̺/ f̺/ v̺/;
- Nasal fricatives /m̥^{F}/ /m/ /n̥^{F}/ /n/ŋ̊^{F}/ŋ/;
- Weak or lax articulation /f͉/ /s͉/ /p͉/ etc.

PRDS recommends that the diacritic [~] is used to denote nasal resonance or escape. ^{F} above a symbol denotes turbulent egressive nasal air-flow eg. /m̥^{F}/.

Phonetic Analysis

Where phonetic production is disordered, careful note should be made of when manner has been preserved, but place has been changed and vice versa. Manner does not often present a problem in the production of nasals, liquids and glides, but plosives, fricatives and affricates are particularly vulnerable, especially in cases where velopharyngeal closure is inadequate.

Any changes in place of articulation should be recorded. Glottal may be used liberally. In some instances double articulation may be used, for example both at the glottis and lips for /p/b/; the glottal stop may be the sound which dominates auditorially, indicating that it is difficult for the individual to get air pressure forward to the lips. The backward shift of articulatory placement in the mouth is frequently found in the speech of individuals with cleft palate.

In evaluation of phonetic abilities all the phonotactic possibilities of a given language should be explored. This may be particularly useful in providing indicators for achieving phonetic changes.

Phonological Analysis

Following the phonetic investigation a phonological analysis should be carried out, using the procedure preferred by the clinician for the analysis of child speech (see **Elbert & Gierut**, 1986 and **Grunwell**, 1985). This level of analysis will establish whether or not the child is able to signal phonological contrasts and whether the limitations are due to inability to produce sounds at the phonetic level. Any phonetic limitations overlap into the phonological level of language. Children will also be passing through the normal processes of phonological development and it is therefore necessary to identify which features are part of phonological development and which are symptomatic of difficulties at articulatory and phonetic levels.

Additional Factors Related to Speech Assessment

Hearing and Auditory Perceptual Skills

Speech evaluation should be accompanied by a thorough evaluation of hearing acuity with referral to the audiologist if indicated. The auditory skills of attention, recognition, discrimination and memory should also be evaluated, as they are essential for the reception and production of speech. The Goldman–Fristoe Auditory Skills Battery may be used (**Goldman *et al***, 1970).

The careful examination of the peripheral speech mechanism, together with a detailed analysis of speech, is essential because the findings obtained form the basis of a precise account of the presenting problem, thus leading to a diagnostic statement and the planning of management and treatment.

CHAPTER 4
HOW CAN THE TEAM HELP?

The Parents / *40*
The Whole Team / *40*
The Plastic Surgeon / *41*
Referrals / *42*
Dental Specialists / *44*
The Orthodontist / *45*
The Prosthetic Specialist / *45*
Oral Surgeon / *45*
Ear, Nose and Throat Surgeon, Audiologist and Teacher of the Deaf / *46*
Radiologist/Radiographer / *47*
The Value of Referrals / *49*

CHAPTER 4
HOW CAN THE TEAM HELP?

Findings from the examination of the peripheral speech mechanism together with the detailed description of speech may present the clinician with a number of questions. The answer to some of these can only be sought through referral to other members of the team. It is therefore important to know:

1 When referral should be made;
2 Who referral should be made to;
3 What information or management the specialist is likely to provide;
4 What information should be made available at referral.

The suggestions made in this chapter are intended for the general clinician. The clinician working in a specialist unit as a member of the cleft palate team may function in somewhat different ways and will, for example, undertake regular clinics with team members. It is hoped that specialist colleagues based in units will act in an advisory capacity to clinicians carrying a general case load, perhaps offering advice concerning clinical medical specialists who have a particular interest and expertise in dealing with the management of conditions associated with cleft lip and palate.

The number of potential members of the cleft palate team is extensive. However, for the adequate management of any individual case, the required group may be quite small. There are always decisions to be made which need a multidisciplinary approach.

The Parents

It is necessary to stress that parents are essential team members, from the traumatic beginnings to adulthood. **Phillips & Stengelhofen** (1989) explored the feelings of parents and made numerous suggestions as to ways in which the clinician might foster parent–professional relationships. Clinicians may have a particular role here, because where there is a speech problem they and the family are likely to have frequent and close contact, giving the opportunity for a relationship which can provide links with and support to the work of the team. Various team members may have significance at different stages of a child's development.

The Whole Team

Figure 4.1 illustrates the involvement of team members at stages of development of the client and indicates when and for how long team members are most likely to be involved. Several team members may be

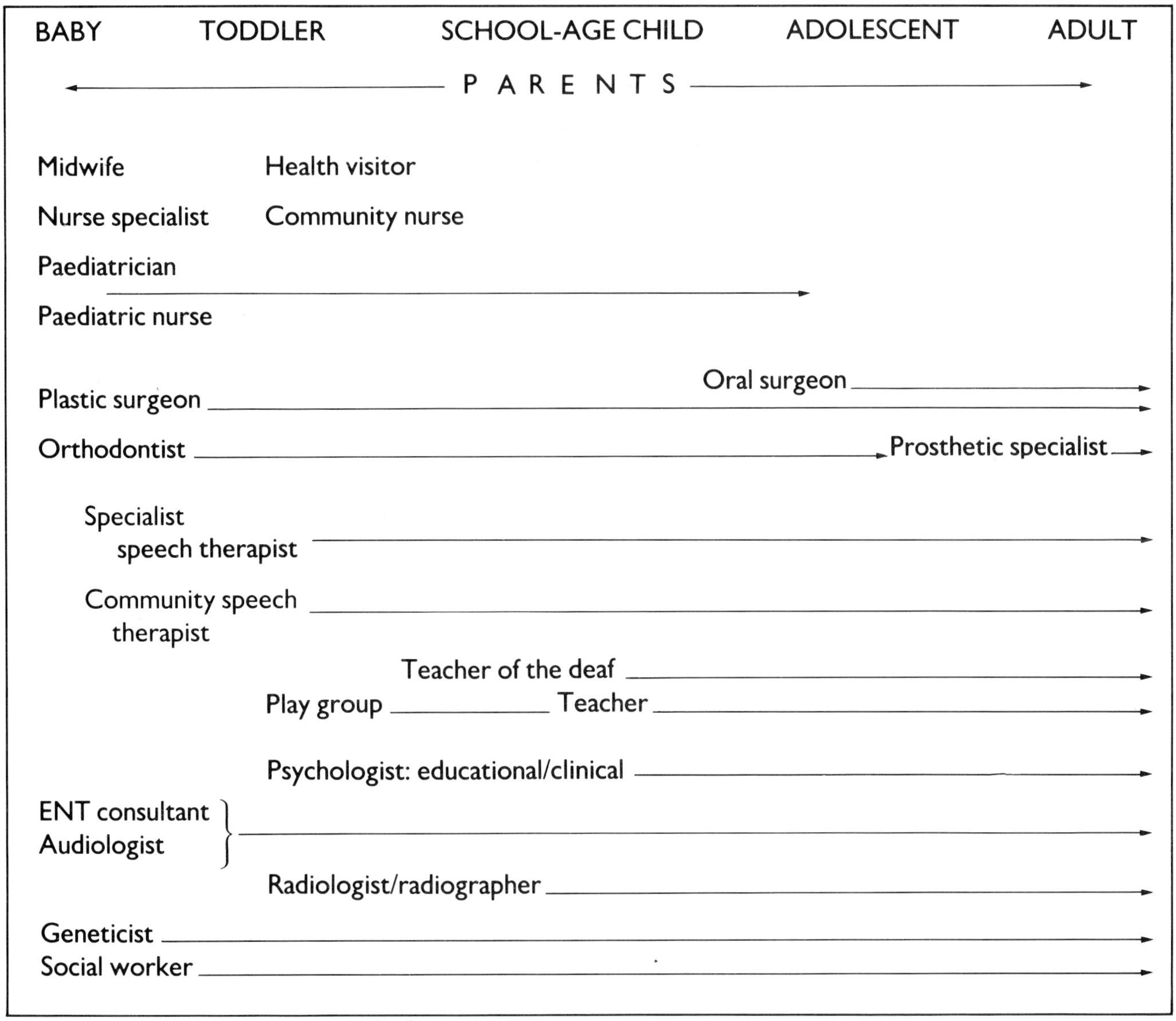

Figure 4.1 ***Team involvement***

involved in aspects of management throughout a child's life and even into adulthood. Clinicians will be concerned with the identification and remediation of communication problems in toddlers, school-age children, adolescents and adults, but are unlikely to be involved in the post-natal period and early infancy unless working in a specialist unit. Children are frequently referred too late and, realistically, the clinician should be involved before the first birthday in monitoring the baby's pre-linguistic skills and in counselling parents. This is a role which can be undertaken by the speech clinician working in general practice (*see Chapter 7*). It is essential that, in the management of individuals with cleft lip and palate, clinicians make full use of the diagnostic and management provisions available from the team.

The Plastic Surgeon

The plastic surgeon is responsible for planning and implementing the surgical intervention for the cleft lip and palate, as well as other conditions involving velopharyngeal incompetence. Surgical procedures for the following are provided:

1 Primary repair of the lip and/or palate, including sub-mucous cleft.
2 Secondary surgery to lip.

3 Secondary surgery to the nose, both to improve the airway and to improve appearance.

4 Secondary surgery to improve the velopharyngeal mechanism in cases of repaired cleft palate.

5 Primary surgery in cases of congenital velopharyngeal incompetence, eg. palatal push-back, pharyngoplasty.

6 Closure of oro-nasal fistula.

Individual surgeons have preferred procedures and times for carrying out primary repairs of cleft lip and palate. Procedures for improvement of the velopharyngeal mechanism need to be tailored to the individual's anatomy. This is now possible through the use of *endoscopic examination* (*see below*).

Referrals

The initial referral to the clinician may well have come from the plastic surgeon. Referrals should be viewed as a two-way process, referring back to the plastic surgeon where the speech findings and/or progress indicate that there is need for further investigation and possibly surgery. On no account should treatment commence if, in the light of assessment, treatment is contraindicated. *Intervention should not proceed if the status of the velopharyngeal mechanism is unknown and the speech manifestations sug-*

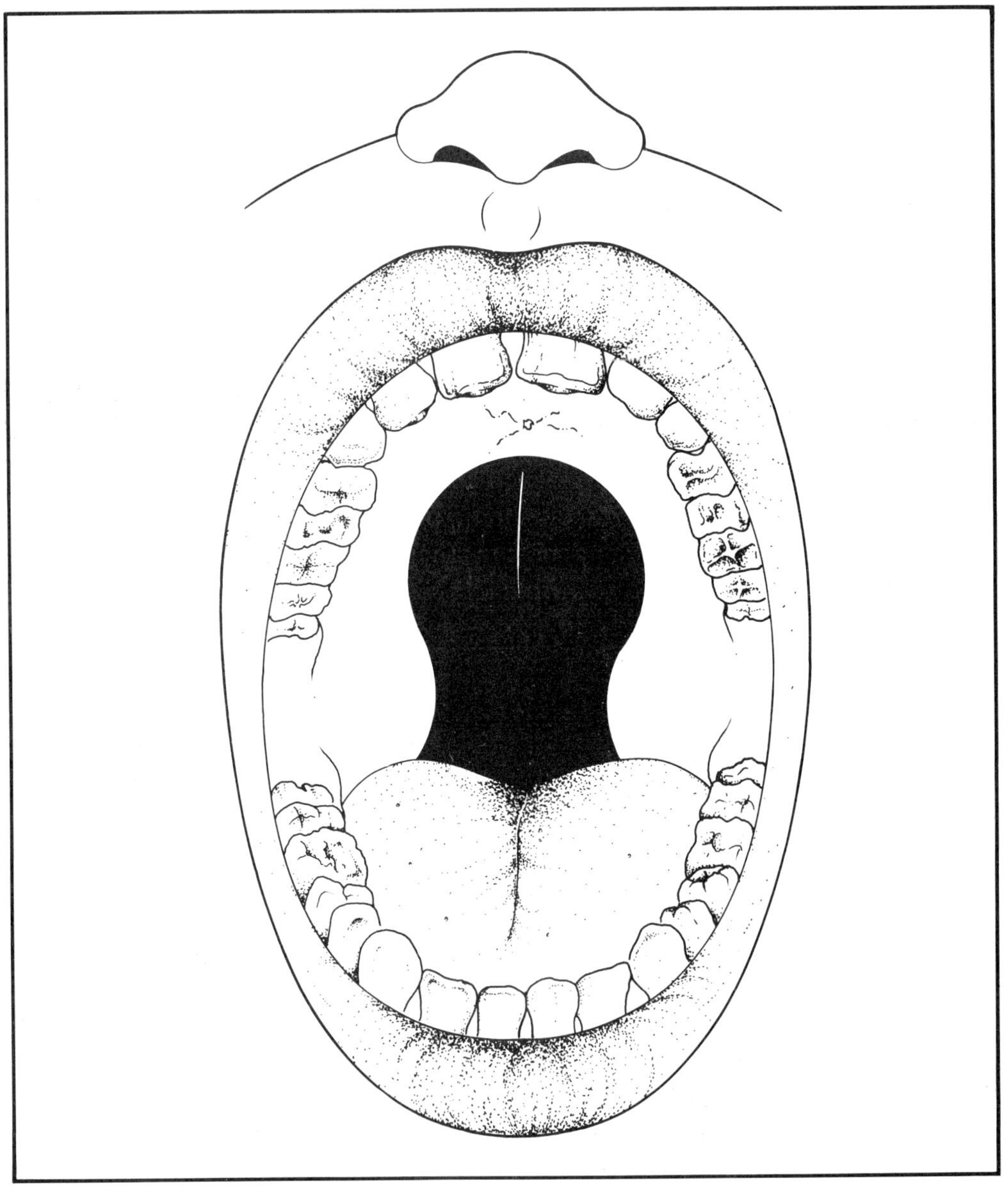

Figure 4.2 ***'U'-shaped cleft***

gest that the mechanism is inadequate. In this situation referral should be made to the plastic surgeon for further investigations. With pre-school children, the use of endoscopic procedures will not be possible, although multiview videofluoroscopy could be a useful alternative.

Referral to the plastic surgeon should be made if speech assessment and examination of the peripheral speech mechanism indicate that there are structural problems causing the speech difficulties. The speech clinician may sometimes be the first to spot signs of a sub-mucous cleft, and will usually be the first to recognise features indicative of velopharyngeal incompetence. In these cases thorough investigations, followed by surgery, if indicated, should ideally precede speech remediation.

There will be some cases which present long-term management problems for the team. Of note are those children who are unable to undergo surgery for palatal cleft, for example in Pierre Robin syndrome, where the cleft is so wide that the surgical outcome is not likely to be satisfactory. (A large 'U'-shaped characteristic cleft is illustrated in *Figure 4.2*.) A further reason to delay palate repair is the presence of a heart defect. Both the plastic surgeon and the clinician face long-term management problems in these cases, the surgeon trying to decide the optimum time for surgery and the clinician hoping that surgery will be undertaken as quickly as possible. Team members need to keep in touch so that there can be a sharing of the problems faced. Parents will also need support in understanding why surgery is being delayed, as well as in coming to terms with and handling the child's severe limitations in speech progress. If the child reaches school age and the palate is still unrepaired, the possible psychosocial and educational consequences need careful monitoring. The clinician can provide an important link between medical and educational provision. Management of the child with a condition such as Pierre Robin syndrome is illustrated in *Figure 4.3*.

The child with Klippel Feil syndrome also has features which present

FEATURES OF SYNDROME

Small lower jaw
Low tongue attachment
Small mouth opening
Midline cleft of palate; usually extensive 'U'-shaped cleft
Occasional tongue tie
Heart defect in some cases

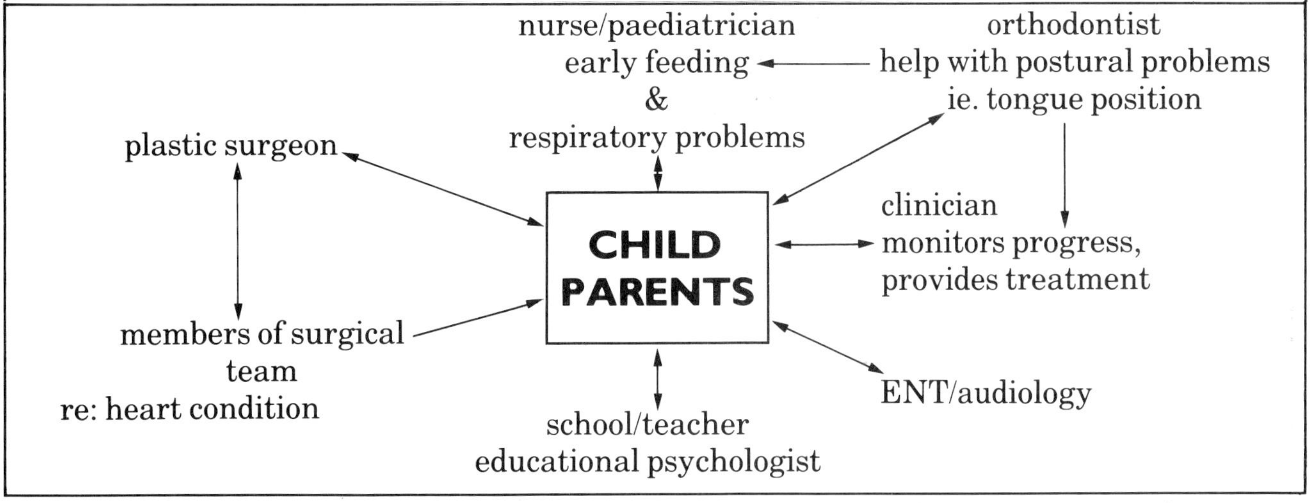

Figure 4.3 ***Management of child with Pierre Robin syndrome***

long-term management problems, as surgery may not be possible because of the lack of neck extension and limited mouth opening. These children will be further disadvantaged in their speech development as a result of impaired hearing, which is characteristic of the syndrome (*see Figure 4.4*). For further accounts of syndromes see **Gorlin *et al*** (1976); **McWilliams *et al*** (1984) and **Travis** (1971).

MAIN FEATURES
Fusion of cervical vertebrae: leads to short neck with restricted head movement. Hairline extends to shoulders. Trapezius muscle flares from mastoid to shoulders.
ADDITIONAL FEATURES
Hearing loss. Cleft palate. Facial asymmetry, possibly with malocclusion.
Note: It is mainly when the additional features are present that there is a major handicap to communication. Palatal repair may not be possible because of restricted head extension and mouth opening. The psychological reactions to the physical impairments may also be significant in relation to the development of communication.

Figure 4.4 ***Features of Klippel Feil syndrome***

A summary of indicators for referral to/back to the plastic surgeon is shown in *Figure 4.5*.

1	Adverse reaction to appearance in older children indicates need for cosmetic revision of nose or lip.
2	Initial speech evaluation in case of repaired cleft palate indicates that the VP mechanism is not adequate.
3	Speech assessment in individuals without history of cleft indicates that there is a problem with the VP mechanism.
4	A diagnostic period of speech intervention has not been successful and supports the hypothesis that VP closure cannot be achieved.
5	Hyponasality and the observation of a crooked nose suggests that a deflected septum may be causing nasal blockage.
6	Evidence that an oro-nasal fistula is the source of nasal emission.
7	Where a palate is unrepaired, eg. Pierre Robin syndrome, there should be regular discussion with the plastic surgeon on the possible timing of surgery.

Figure 4.5 ***Indications for referral to plastic surgeon***

Dental Specialists

In addition to dentists carrying out routine dental treatment the orthodontist and/or prosthetic specialist may also be involved in the management of individuals with cleft lip and/or palate.

The Orthodontist

The orthodontist is involved in making provision for the alignment of the dento-alveolar and maxillary and mandibular structures. The orthodontist may be involved with the individual with cleft lip and/or palate throughout many stages of development. There are three key stages for intervention:

1 From birth to primary surgical repair of lip and alveolus in order to:
   (a) carry out pre-surgical alignment of the upper jaw structures, including the provision of strapping for the lip;
   (b) provide feeding plates;
   (c) provide cradles for babies who are at risk of the tongue blocking the air way (Pierre Robin syndrome).

2 Mixed dentition phase in order to:
   (a) correct incisor positions;
   (b) advise the family and team on growth factors which need to be taken into consideration by the team in planning intervention;
   (c) provide obturators in unrepaired clefts or for oro-nasal fistula;
   (d) monitor and advise on oral hygiene in order to maintain dentition.

3 Permanent dentition phase in order to:
   (a) remove teeth, eg. crowding or supernumerary;
   (b) align molars or incisors;
   (c) correct arch form;
   (d) provide obturators for unrepaired cleft palate;
   (e) provide obturators for oro-nasal fistula;
   (f) provide dentures for missing incisors etc;
   (g) provide plates to be used with PTA, VSA and EPG (electropalatography) (*see Chapter 9*);
   (h) monitor and advise on oral hygiene — of major importance for individuals who receive orthodontic intervention or are long-term appliance wearers.

Prosthetic provisions may be made by the orthodontist or prosthetic specialist. New adult referrals will usually be to the prosthetic specialist, while an orthodontist who has worked with a case from infancy may well continue with that case at least into young adulthood.

The Prosthetic Specialist

The prosthetic specialist tends to be involved more with the older patient, in the replacement of dental and other oral structures, making major contributions to the cosmetic, masticatory and speech aspects of management, both in cases of cleft lip and palate and other conditions where a prosthesis may be required. Older patients with unrepaired cleft palates are likely to be under the care of the prosthetic specialist. Clinicians and prosthetic specialists may also need to work together in the management of cases with acquired neurological disorders which affect the soft palate or pharynx. *Figure 4.6* indicates where referral should be made to a dental specialist.

Oral Surgeon

The oral surgeon works in conjunction with dental colleagues. Referral to the oral surgeon should therefore only be made in consultation with the plastic surgeon and dental specialists concerned with the case. Oral surgery may be recommended where a malocclusion persists into adolescence and remains so severe that it is a handicap to appearance, mastication and communication. Individuals with a Class III malocclusion or oro-nasal fistula are the most likely client groups requiring referral to the oral surgeon.

If plastic surgeons are not keen to operate on oro-nasal fistulae, the oral surgeon may become involved. Fistula repair is sometimes carried out alongside other oral surgery procedures. The oral surgeon will liaise with the plastic surgeon. All team members, together with the individual concerned, need to be included in the discussions about the need for surgical intervention.

1	Malocclusions.
2	Anterior open bite.
3	Oro-nasal fistula; to provide temporary obturation to establish the significance in speech, or permanent obturation where the significance has been established and surgery is not recommended. A number of cleft cases will be permanent denture wearers.
4	Provision of obturator in unrepaired cleft.
5	Provision of plates to be used with VSA, PTA and EPG.

Figure 4.6 ***Indications for referral to dental specialist***

Ear, Nose and Throat Surgeon, Audiologist and Teacher of the Deaf

The frequent occurrence of hearing loss in cases of cleft palate was discussed in *Chapter 1*. Hearing impairment in infants as early as age three months has been noted. The ENT specialist is therefore likely to be involved early on in the medical and surgical management of middle-ear disease. The management of hearing is of vital importance to the development of normal communication as well as to the remediation of communication problems. Myringotomies and grommet insertions are frequently undertaken.

The fluctuating nature of the hearing impairment means that it will need to be checked regularly; a frequency of every three to six months may be necessary when hearing is not stable. If the child is seen on a regular basis, a close watch can be kept on the hearing status through general observation, reports from parents and school and from the use of screening audiometry. Auditory discrimination procedures such as in the Goldman–Fristoe Auditory Skills Battery may also be used as a screening procedure. The clinician can play a valuable role in:

1 Alerting teachers to the presence of hearing loss, especially of the fluctuating nature;

2 Advising on classroom seating;

3 Advising on the importance of the use of the visual channel to aid the auditory;

4 Advising on the care of hearing-aids.

The audiologist will be involved in complex assessments of auditory function, such as:

1 Pure tone audiometry, including the evaluation of the air-bone gap;
2 Speech audiometry — to assess the functional use of hearing for speech and for evaluation of the suitability of a hearing-aid;
3 Procedures to evaluate the function of the middle ear, such as impedance audiometry;
4 Free field and play audiometry procedures with young children;
5 Distraction tests.

Middle-ear disease may be caused and maintained through hypertrophied adenoids. However, as the adenoids may also be involved in achieving velopharyngeal closure, the ENT surgeon is not likely to remove these without consulting the plastic surgeon as to the possible effect their removal might have on the velopharyngeal mechanism. Where adenoidectomy is essential for the improvement of middle-ear function a procedure can be used where only lateral elements of the adenoids, nearest the Eustachian Tube, are removed.

There is controversy over the view that hypertrophied tonsils may rest on the velum, push it down and forward and cause more nasality (**Morris**, 1975). This factor should be taken into account in the assessment of velopharyngeal function.

The maintenance of a good relationship with the ENT specialist should ensure that the advisability of surgical procedures and their relation to possible speech outcomes are jointly considered. In cases where severe phonatory changes are evident, referral should be made to the ENT specialist to explore the status of the larynx through either direct or indirect laryngoscopy. It may occasionally be possible for nasendoscopy and laryngoscopy to be carried out concurrently. The management of identified vocal fold nodules will need careful consideration early on in the treatment plan.

ENT surgeons may occasionally refer children when hypernasality persists post-adenoidectomy. The status of the velopharyngeal mechanism needs to be established and management planned on the basis of the findings. Speech therapy is contraindicated if the anatomical proportions do not have the potential for velopharyngeal closure. Consultation between ENT surgeon, clinician, plastic surgeon and radiologist needs to take place in deciding an appropriate management plan.

Some children with severe degrees of hearing impairment will be receiving help either pre-school or at school age from a teacher of the deaf. It is essential that the clinician and teacher of the deaf meet to explore the nature of the speech, language and learning difficulties with which they are both concerned. Ideally a joint intervention plan should be developed, with regular joint review of progress. The clinician can provide the teacher of the deaf with information on the nature of speech problems associated with the cleft palate condition, so that the appropriateness of various intervention procedures for speech can be considered. *Figure 4.7* indicates when referral should be made to the ENT consultant and audiologist.

Radiologist/Radiographer

The role of the radiologist is to aid the diagnosis of abnormal structure and function. **Huskie** (1989) provides a full account of how the team work together in arriving at an objective account of the function of the velopharyngeal mechanism. The radiologist has a central role to play in this. It is

1	Need for full audiological assessment when initial observations and screening suggest hearing impairment.
2	Hypertrophied tonsils and adenoids.
3	Persistent hyponasality and other speech features associated with nasal blockage.
4	Persistent hypernasality following adenoidectomy.
5	Need for laryngeal examination in phonatory disorders.
6	Nasendoscopy.

Figure 4.7 ***Indications for referral to ENT consultant/audiologist***

usually within the specialist cleft palate unit that the procedures are undertaken, using the skills, expertise and equipment which are available in such a setting. Clinicians in general practice will find that they can learn a great deal from attending appointments with patients when diagnostic procedures are undertaken.

Where there is doubt regarding the adequacy of the velopharyngeal mechanism, a request should be made, normally through the plastic surgeon, for further investigations. In making the referral it is advisable to name the procedures which are requested. The procedures most likely to be available are:

1 *Speech radiography*: the clinician will be able to assess the child's potential for co-operation in keeping the head still and speaking on request. The speech clinician working regularly with the child may be the best person to elicit data, rather than the clinician working in the specialist unit.
2 *Lateral radiographs*: this is a limited procedure, as the view only includes lateral aspects of the velopharyngeal mechanism and does not include movement in speech.
3 *Cineradiography*: provides a view of the structures in speech and swallowing.
4 *Multiview videofluoroscopy*: a diagnostic procedure to look at the function of the velopharyngeal mechanism.

In addition to the procedures involving radiography, the development of *nasendoscopic examination* provides the most comprehensive picture of the function of the velopharyngeal mechanism. This may be carried out either by the plastic surgeon or the ENT surgeon and the clinician. Nasendoscopy is fully described by **Huskie** (1989) and **Pigott** (1980). Again this is a procedure which can be helped by the presence of the clinician who knows the child. It is not likely that it can be undertaken with pre-school children, although Pigott mentions children of three years of age who 'responded without apparent fear'.

The technique introduces a flexible or rigid endoscope into an anaesthetised nostril to gain a view looking down onto the velopharyngeal isthmus. The view is displayed on a video screen and video recorded for further analysis. The procedure is invasive and requires careful explanation to the patient or both child and parents. The clinician may be able to support the undertaking of this examination by the provision of careful explanations to child and parent before agreement for referral, and being present to elicit speech data if a young child is reluctant to talk to strangers. Benefit will also be gained by attending the appointment to see the view of the velo-pharyngeal mechanism first-hand.

The Value of Referrals

In making a referral to another specialist be clear about the implications and possible outcomes. The clinician and the team members concerned need to address a number of questions. *Figure 4.8* summarises the process.

1	Evaluation of speech indicates that a problem is present which needs diagnosis and/or management by members of team.
2	Referral is made accompanied by a concise report, giving the findings and indicating how these may relate to the condition in question. (It is advisable to request referral to a named specialist.)
3	Specialist sees case — confirms or rejects.
4	Specialist reports back to the clinician (? via GP).
5	If the condition is confirmed, the team members involved need to address the following questions: (a) Would the treatment (surgery/orthodontics etc) be likely to help speech? (b) How soon can treatment be provided? (c) If there is a delay, should speech therapy continue or be suspended? (d) Will speech therapy be needed after the prescribed treatment? If yes, this needs to be made clear to parents and child. (e) What is the length of the treatment? (f) What is the most likely outcome? (g) Some treatments, eg. orthodontic and speech therapy, can run concurrently; is this indicated?
6	Proceed when all questions have been addressed and ALL concerned, including the parents and child, understand what is involved.

Figure 4.8 ***The process of referral***

With the heavy case load carried by clinicians, as well as the lack of adequate clerical support, it may be difficult to provide the team with reports as frequently as desirable. This aspect of case management is nevertheless extremely important. It is all too easy for some of the team members to reach a decision about a case when other members are not present. It is therefore always advisable to provide a comprehensive report:

1 Following initial speech and language evaluation;

2 At the stage of referral to another agency;

3 When a case is being reviewed by another member of the team.

If these steps are followed clinicians will not find themselves in the position of learning that a decision has been reached without the speech and language status being taken into account in an informed way. This still happens far too frequently and it is often because the clinician working regularly with the case has not submitted a report. Whenever possible, the speech clinician should attend appointments which are of major consequence in case management. Time taken to attend an appointment will save time in the end if it means that appropriate decisions are made. How many of us have heard mothers say, "X says he can carry on with his speech therapy for another year"?

In the above sections the role of some of the potential team members has been outlined. Others who might also be involved were indicated in *Figure 4.1*. The more complex the condition, the more extensive the team is likely to be. In this complexity of team management it is unfortunately only too easy for parents (and patient) to feel overlooked and confused. Indeed they are sometimes on the receiving end of conflicting advice. This no doubt happens unintentionally but is a result of inadequate communication between team members. It is the responsibility of all involved to try to develop a system in which the patient is not lost in the maze. The clinician can participate in and contribute to communication in the team in the following ways:

1. Attend or set up joint clinics if these do not operate.
2. Attend or set up case conferences if these do not operate.
3. Write regular updating reports, with copies to all team members.
4. Establish a central involvement in the team.
5. Support the need for and explain treatments offered by other team members if this is not understood.
6. Help in the care of appliances, eg. orthodontic appliances, hearing-aids.
7. Assist child and parents in understanding procedures to be used by other team members.
8. Take matters raised by patients and carers back to team members.
9. Develop own understanding of the procedures used by others as well as enhancing the appreciation of the limitations and extent of various provisions, through clinic attendance, discussion and reading.
10. Examine speech intervention in the context of total management needs, including the appropriateness of the timing.
11. If unable to attend specialist appointments, ensure that parents are prepared to ask relevant questions.
12. Keep in touch with the speech clinician in the cleft palate unit, who may be able to provide guidance on treatment and on the need for referral.
13. Encourage parents to attend all appointments. Where there are difficulties approach other relevant services, for example social services and voluntary bodies such as the Red Cross or the Women's Royal Voluntary Service (WRVS).

These ideas have been explored further by **Phillips & Stengelhofen** (1989).

CHAPTER 5
PATTERNS OF SPEECH THERAPY PROVISION

Considering the Prognosis / *52*

When Should Speech Intervention Begin? / *52*

The Baby / *52*

The Pre-school Child / *53*

The School-age Child / *54*

Adolescents and Young Adults / *54*

The Older Age Group / *55*

Deferring the Onset of Treatment / *55*

Patterns of Provision / *55*

Intensive and/or Continuing Therapy / *55*

Group or Individual Therapy / *57*

CHAPTER 5
PATTERNS OF SPEECH THERAPY PROVISION

Considering the Prognosis

In undertaking the treatment of communication difficulties in a child, adolescent or adult with cleft palate it is essential to make a careful appraisal of all the factors, in order to make a statement about long-term outcomes. This prognostic statement in relation to speech is essential in setting realistic expectations for the patient, relatives, team and clinician. Prognosis must include advice from the rest of the team, as their management may have a major influence on the speech outcomes.

In taking on a case it is also necessary to make clear to all those involved that the process of intervention may need to take place over an extended period. When working with young children, however, it is important, if clearly warranted, to give the parents a positive view of the outcome in the knowledge that the majority of cases will develop normal speech and language after successful surgery in infancy, without requiring any specific speech intervention. This assumes that no condition exists which is likely to be a handicap to the development of normal speech.

Treatment of communication will need to be co-ordinated with other management provisions. There will be periods when, for example, speech intervention is not carried out because surgery is awaited, while at other times speech remediation needs to be the priority. Where a child and family are involved, in many forms of treatment, they will sometimes find it difficult to maintain their motivation. In the interests of the successful long-term outcome, the child's and the family's feelings and views need to be taken into account, because their involvement in and motivation towards bringing about change is essential.

Figure 5.1 suggests a list of factors which need to be considered in arriving at a prognostic statement. *Appendix II* provides a proforma to complete in arriving at this statement. Each item included in the statement should be an area which has been discussed fully with the parents, the child (if at an appropriate age) or the adult patient. Each item should be evaluated on the six-point scale.

When Should Speech Intervention Begin?

The Baby

The clinician should be involved very early on in the management of the baby with cleft palate. When the clinician works in a specialist unit it will be possible for the first contact to take place before operative procedures to the palate, so that there is opportunity to discuss speech and language develop-

1	Nature and severity of original condition.
2	Age at initial surgery to palate.
3	Plans for surgery if not already undertaken.
4	Success of operation in terms of velopharyngeal mechanism/ fistula etc.
5	Status of vocal tract, including dental and occlusal factors.
6	Status of larynx.
7	State of speech and language development at primary and secondary operations.
8	Hearing.
9	Intellectual factors.
10	Emotional adjustment of individual in general and to communication in particular.
11	The presence of any other handicapping physical conditions, such as found in some syndromes.
12	Availability and efficacy of provisions, including speech therapy.
13	Motivation of individual towards communication changes.
14	Family support and adjustment.

Figure 5.1 ***Factors affecting eventual speech and language outcomes***

ment with the parents and how this may be encouraged, whether or not surgery is to proceed. The function of the palate in speech should be explained. The plastic surgeon should give a realistic picture for the operative outcomes. Initially the role of the clinician should focus on monitoring progress, the evaluation of speech and language, and counselling. With contact established and regular monitoring undertaken, more specific intervention procedures can be initiated as necessary. Ways of working with the baby and the pre-school child will be discussed in detail in *Chapter 7*.

The Pre-school Child

It is an ideal aim to enable all children to enter school with adequate communication. The pre-school period is therefore a key time for remediating speech (*see Chapter 7*). Specific intervention for speech should begin in the pre-school years, if the following questions have a positive answer:

1 Has the palatal repair been undertaken? In some instances where surgery is not possible it may be possible to start some pre-speech work (*see Chapter 7*).
2 Is the result to the palatal repair such that the achievement of velopharyngeal closure seems likely?
3 Is the child mature enough to co-operate at some level, in particular with the parents who will be carrying out the day-to-day work?
4 Are the parents motivated about working with their child?
5 Do the parents understand and accept their role in undertaking the regular work with their child?

Intervention at this time may be carried out in the specialist unit, but should ideally be undertaken in the child's home locality, where it will relate to other provisions such as are offered by the health visitor, play group etc.

The School-age Child

If the child is first referred at school age, management must begin with a careful evaluation of the oral and velopharyngeal structures and the analysis of speech and language. If there is any doubt about the adequacy of the velopharyngeal mechanism, referral should be made for full investigation (plastic surgeon and radiologist; *see Chapter 4*).

If the mechanism for speech is inadequate, intervention for speech may be contraindicated, as this may encourage the child to attempt to articulate in ways which are not physically possible and may precipitate or exacerbate deviant patterns.

Where delay in language development has been found, intervention focused on language development should proceed. Discussion should take place with school staff about how they view the child's communication and how language development may be promoted in school. The particular needs of children with hearing impairment should be considered.

Speech and language intervention for the school-age child should be viewed as a priority in case management. If speech problems are found in a child and the velopharyngeal mechanism is considered to be adequate, intervention should proceed. The possible patterns of provision are outlined below. In some instances a school-age child will be referred who does not have an overt cleft palate but presents features of:

HYPERNASALITY — with possible nasal emission and nasal grimace.

ARTICULATORY PROBLEMS — especially poor or weakened fricatives and/or plosives.

PHONATORY PROBLEMS — possibly drooling or facial weakness.

Speech intervention should not be undertaken with such children until the status of the velopharyngeal mechanism is established.

Adolescents and Young Adults

Where communication problems persist into adolescence and adulthood, remediation needs extremely careful planning. The standard of speech should be measured against the adequacy and acceptability of communication and not against some theoretical 'normal' standard. The range of acceptability is wide, varying with an individual's needs and expectations. Where young people have other handicapping conditions it will be important to bring all the services together in trying to improve communication skills, which are crucially important in social adjustment and the ability to gain employment.

The evaluation of the adequacy of the velopharyngeal mechanism is of central importance. Other factors, such as malocclusion or hearing loss, will need management. Adolescents and young adults must be fully involved in bringing about their own speech and communication changes and will need to be made aware at the outset of the time commitment and personal effort required. Sometimes young people request help on their own account where the history has been one of inconsistent attendance and poor family support. Where self-motivation is evident, further treatment should be provided. A contract should be entered into which includes a clearly defined trial period of treatment.

The drawing-up of a contract helps all participants to understand the nature, goals, possible outcomes and their part in the treatment process. A clear agreement about the time provides clinicians and clients with an opportunity to review progress objectively. With adolescents and older clients and parents of young children the contract can help to provide the motivation to carry out the hard work necessary to achieve change.

The Older Age Group

Occasionally individuals in middle life seek help with their speech. They may have an unrepaired or poorly repaired cleft palate, or be undiagnosed cases of CPI. Sometimes, when an obturator or new dentures are being fitted, clients may ask if there is any help available for their speech. In other instances social or employment factors may put pressure on them to improve their communication (*see the case of Mr N in Chapter 10*).

Surgery to improve an inadequate mechanism may not be an appropriate option. In cases of unrepaired cleft palate the fitting of an obturator with an extension into the velopharyngeal area should be considered with the prosthetic specialist. The clinician can provide an objective evaluation of the effect of different appliances on speech.

Some adults are so highly motivated to improve their speech that they make remarkable progress in the context of the inadequacy of the mechanism. Be cautious and realistic about the possible outcomes of therapy, but be willing to enter into a trial period of treatment on a contractual basis. If surgery is to take place, the possible consequences for speech need full and realistic exploration. This aspect may not have been handled comprehensively by the plastic surgeon, so check the patient's expectations.

Adolescents and adults with seemingly entrenched speech problems may be helped by the use of instrumental procedures. PTA and VSA may be used when the palate is repaired. Electropalatography may provide the essential visual feedback in helping to modify articulatory placements (*see Chapter 9*).

Deferring the Onset of Treatment

It is always better to delay the start of treatment than to begin and make no progress, or have disappointing results. This is demotivating for the patient, the carers and the clinician. *Figure 5.2* summarises the factors which might indicate that treatment should be deferred.

Patterns of Provision

With many developmental speech and language problems it is essential to make provision when the child is first seen and to continue until such time as there is a satisfactory outcome or the maximum potential is reached. In individuals with cleft palate, because of the possible long-term nature of the problem, the pattern in which the treatment is delivered needs particular consideration. Treatment should be tailored to the individual needs of each child, the family, the nature of the condition and the associated handicapping conditions.

Intensive and/or Continuing Therapy

There will be initial involvement with babies and toddlers in a monitoring and a counselling capacity. This may only need to be on an occasional basis,

1	When the status of the velopharyngeal mechanism is not established, unless the speech intervention is part of the diagnostic process.
2	Operative procedures are imminent.
3	Immediately post-operative, when the palate and/or pharynx may be oedematous and stiff.
4	Patient motivation is lacking.
5	If parent support is not available, alternative management should be explored.
6	Child is not mature enough to co-operate with specific work.
7	Where some other form of management needs to take precedence at a particular time.
8	Waiting for the provision of an aid which is considered to be an essential adjunct to treatment, eg. hearing-aid, PTA.
9	Child has just begun school/new school and needs a settling-in period.
10	Intensive therapy at school age needs to be arranged at an appropriate age for the child.
Note: Some authorities believe that articulation therapy should precede pharyngoplasty, when velopharyngeal closure cannot be achieved.	

Figure 5.2 ***Delaying speech intervention***

the baby or toddler being seen when attending for other appointments — perhaps with the paediatrician or plastic surgeon. A model for initial contacts of the speech clinician with the parents is described by **Russell** (1989).

In some countries there is a tendency to provide treatment regimes on a weekly basis. In many instances the speech clinician only attends a clinic on such a basis, placing major constraints on the way a service can be delivered. With young children where work at an articulatory level is required, intervention once a week, even with the parents carrying out regular work in between appointments, may not be sufficient to change patterns already laid down. To break into these patterns something more intensive may be required, at least initially, after which a different regime, concentrating on maintenance and generalisation, may be adopted. A flexible regime needs to be adopted where the pattern of provision can easily move from intensive to less frequent to longer periods of stabilisation.

With school-age children it is unwise to enter into a weekly treatment regime which seems to have no end for all concerned. Short bouts of intervention, interspersed with periods of stabilisation, are likely to be much more productive and motivating for child, family and clinician and may well be less disruptive to schooling.

The clinician responsible for the case needs to recognise that other clinicians can contribute to the treatment. A small team of therapists can work effectively together on speech, having set up agreed aims precisely directed at the problems identified. Initial assessment is probably best carried out by one clinician. By working in this way it might be possible to provide a child or adult with daily help for a short period. School holiday time can be used productively, especially where children miss a lot of schooling because of numerous appointments for many aspects of their condition.

Studies in the efficacy of intensive therapy (**Albery & Enderby**, 1984; **Huskie**, 1979 and **Van Demark & Hardin**, 1986) show some of the advantages of intensive as well as residential treatment. It is recognised that health authorities may not be able to set up residential provision, the desirability of which is open to debate. However departments may be able to follow similar models, where intensive periods offered in one centre may be followed by more extended work in the patient's own locality.

Group or Individual Therapy

The intensive treatment regimes referred to above also involve working with children in pairs or in small groups. This is another factor which might be significant in relation to progress and one that should be considered as part of case management. It is unlikely that one therapist in a locality will have a suitable group of children with cleft palate, but a group could be collected across localities. Group work could take place on a weekly basis or be the pattern of provision for an intensive course on a daily basis. There are a number of advantages in arranging group therapy. The following are suggested:

1. Clinicians may be involved who have a special interest in these conditions, so that their expertise is used to full effect.
2. If a group is of a size to need two clinicians (other professional or helper or student) more creative treatment ideas are likely to be generated.
3. Children may fit more easily into a group if they feel pressure in the one-to-one situation.
4. Children may learn from each other.
5. Functional communication can be more easily observed, evaluated and improved.
6. Excellent opportunities are provided for work on such areas as auditory skill development.
7. Children can, if necessary, be taken aside for a short period of individual help.
8. A wide range of opportunities is provided for transfer of new skills and generalisation into everyday speech.
9. Opportunities to talk are ensured. Some children may not talk in school.
10. Language work can easily be integrated.
11. Children may receive psychological support from meeting others with similar difficulties.
12. The involvement of parents in group work enhances their understanding of the nature of the difficulties and of the helping process.
13. The meeting of parents can provide mutual support.

Group and intensive therapy may be provided in school holiday periods. Clinicians working in schools may be more easily available at such times and do not have to cancel routine commitments. Children do not miss schooling. The difficulties of setting up a cohesive group, providing transport and suitable accommodation are fully recognised.

Chapter 6
General Principles of Intervention

CHAPTER 6
GENERAL PRINCIPLES OF INTERVENTION

Principles of intervention vary to some extent according to the age and needs of the individual and the constraints of any handicapping condition. Generally the following principles should stand:

1 Be involved early on in decisions about general case management; *no age is too young*.

2 Give explanations to the parents/carers on the nature of the provision, ie treatment, counselling, monitoring etc.

3 The individuals concerned, plus parents or carers, should be motivated towards the provision being offered.

4 The intervention plan must be clearly aimed at the particular problems identified through detailed assessment.

5 Adopt a pattern of provision which is most likely to achieve a successful outcome for the individual.

6 Decide the long- and short-term goals; normal speech may not be one of them. Ideally the goal should be for the *acquisition of speech which is acceptable to the individual and the social environment.*

7 When a child is of an age to understand, simple explanations should be provided about the problems and what is to be done to help. The child may already be aware of poor speech and appearance.

8 Use as many sensory approaches in treatment as possible, ie tactile, visual, auditory.

9 Consider the use of mechanical aids in the provision of feedback:

- Mirror;
- Relaxometer;
- 'N' indicator (*see* **Stuffins**, 1989);
- Training plate with ridges/grooves;
- PTA and VSA;
- Visi-speech;
- Electropalatography.

(*See Chapter 9.*)

10 The programme should be graded in very small steps so as to ensure success.

11 Start with an area where there is likely to be success, rather than necessarily working on an aspect where difficulties may be more obvious.

12 With adolescents, adults and parents, help them to achieve as much insight as possible into the nature of the speech/language difficulties, their causes and suggested management.

13 Consider ways to maintain motivation and increase insight into improvement through progress charts, rating scales, diaries etc.

14 In planning intervention include objectives related to:

(a) specific features of speech, eg. phonatory/articulatory;

(b) more general communication factors, eg. rate of utterance/volume.

In this way the communication improvement will be approached from different angles, and all possibilities of achieving change will be explored.

15 Attention to features such as volume, rate and prosody may play as important a part in improving intelligibility as working on the articulation.

16 With the older child and adult adopt methods of treatment presentation which are likely to be acceptable, eg. prepared tape work, diagrams, self-rating scales, use of instrumentation.

17 There should be open discussion of the physical condition with the individual concerned as well as parents or carers.

18 *If the soft palate is not long enough to reach the pharyngeal wall, no amount of exercise will get it there.*

19 *Never allow the individual child or adult to do anything in speaking which leads to excessive effort.* The vocal tract is a dynamic apparatus. Excessive tension in one area will have undesirable overflow effects. Any increase in tension will exacerbate unwanted features such as audible nasal emission, glottalisation and vocal abuse.

20 Blowing and sucking exercises, are *not* found to be effective in improving the function of the velopharyngeal mechanism in speech, therefore they should not be used. The playing of wind instruments and using blowing toys are also usually contraindicated because they are likely to require effortful blowing and will exacerbate nasal grimace and turbulence. If nasal passages and nares become restricted by the physical effort, the audibility of the nasal air-flow will increase.

21 The treatment plan for speech must include work on simple production, eg. in consonant/vowel (CV) combinations, working up to complex combinations to include all the phonotactic possibilities of a given language, to words, sentences, connected prepared speech and to spontaneous speech.

22 During intervention there should be frequent evaluation of the efficacy of the intervention, as well as a reconsideration of the adequacy of the physical mechanisms. Sometimes it will be necessary to set up a period of diagnostic therapy in order to establish whether or not the individual is able to improve, for example if there is uncertainty about the adequacy of the velopharyngeal mechanism. It may not be possible to carry out a diagnostic procedure such as nasendoscopy. Speech intervention will be used as part of the diagnostic process. Another instance would be where it is difficult to decide whether an oro-nasal fistula or the velopharyngeal mechanism is the source of nasal emission and associated reduced intra-oral air pressure. **Albery** (1989), suggests three to six months' diagnostic therapy.

23 A period of diagnostic therapy must be precisely directed at an objective which will help to establish the hypothesis set: eg. X is able to achieve velopharyngeal closure. In this case work should be directed to the production of sounds which require a high level of intra-oral air pressure, ie plosives and fricatives. It is not sufficient for these to be achieved in isolation. Newly-acquired sounds must be produced at least in CV combinations and in words with a degree of articulatory ease, at a reasonable speed and not accompanied by hypernasality, nasal escape or nasal grimace.

24 Help individuals build up an ability to monitor their own performance.

25 Both language and speech development and their interrelationship should be fully explored and treated in an integrated way.

26 In working on children's speech it is usually advisable to follow the sequence of normal phonetic and phonological development.

27 Provide appropriate analogies to help the child or adult understand how regular practice is essential for speech improvement; eg. football, dancing, piano.

CHAPTER 7
WORKING WITH BABIES & YOUNG CHILDREN

Early Speech Development in Infants with Cleft Palate / *64*
Ensuring that Speech and Language Follow Expected Development / *64*
Working with Toddlers up to School Age / *69*
Speech or Language Intervention? / *70*
Principles for Specific Work on Speech in Young Children / *72*

CHAPTER 7
WORKING WITH BABIES & YOUNG CHILDREN

Early Speech Development in Infants with Cleft Palate

It is only in recent years that there has been detailed study of the development of vocalisations in infants with cleft palate as well as of the effect of surgery on vocalisations. It has been found that it is not unusual in the case of operative intervention in infancy for the early vocalisations, gained pre-operatively, to reduce in the immediate post-operative period. This reduction is due to oedema, associated discomfort and the psychological impact of hospitalisation and operation. However, providing surgery has been straightforward and all goes well in the post-operative period, vocalisations should gradually return to the pre-operative level, both in quantity and quality, and from there progress towards 'normal' speech and language development (**Grunwell & Russell**, 1987). Studies such as that by Grunwell and Russell also provide objective evidence that, in the babies studied pre-operatively, there were glottals and a few velars, but no plosives in the vocalisations.

Initially parents are generally not particularly concerned about speech, which is understandable in the context of concern about feeding, the baby's appearance and forthcoming operations. However in the post-operative period they gradually become ready to think about speech development.

Ensuring that Speech and Language Follow Expected Development

General measures can be taken to ensure that speech and language follow expected developmental norms. The following approaches are suggested:

1 *Meet the parents before the operation on the palate* in order to establish a supportive relationship and to explain the nature of the cleft palate condition and how it relates to the development of communication. Examining their own oral structures may help them to understand the function of the palate, and why the repair is necessary. Reassure the parents that, if any long-term help is needed, the clinician will be available — if this is true. (The clinician in the specialist unit may be able to see the parents while the baby is in hospital.)

2 *Post-operatively, undertake regular monitoring of speech and language development.* First of all ascertain what the parents understand about cleft lip and palate and how this relates to speech. They may by this time

have gathered a good deal of information, perhaps not all correct. This kind of discussion will also provide insight into the parents' level of understanding of the process of language development in order to form a basis for advice. Hand-outs and leaflets should be provided, such as those supplied in the UK by Cleft Lip and Palate Association (CLAPA), or the College of Speech Therapists (CST), or the booklet prepared by the Cleft Palate Unit at the Frenchay Hospital, Bristol. In the US, information is available through the American Cleft Palate Educational Foundation.

If parents are in agreement, and if they have play-back facilities, it is very useful to audio-record the discussions with them. This recording can then be listened to at home and they can return with their queries. This can be of particular use if only one parent has been present. Grandparents and others in close touch with the baby may also benefit.

Regular monitoring ensures that problems which arise will be quickly recognised and appropriate management arranged. For example, if hearing impairment is noted, referral can be made to the ENT specialist.

3 *Provide counselling support to the parents in relation to their reactions to having a child with an impairment.* Parents having a child with an impairment frequently experience:

- Shock and extreme emotional upset;
- Disbelief and denial;
- Grief;
- Isolation and inability to share feelings;
- Need to blame someone (or something leads to a sense of guilt);
- Shame and embarrassment;
- Over-compensation, leading to over-protection;
- Lowering of self-esteem;
- Lack of confidence;
- Uncertainty in handling. (**Judson & Burden**, 1980.)

Asking parents why they think the baby has a cleft may provide valuable insight into attitudes which may have a strong effect on the ability of the family to cope with and accept available provision. This may be particularly significant where the culture of the family is different from that of the clinician. **Phillips & Stengelhofen** (1989) provide further insight into parents' reactions.

Clinicians can bring counselling skills to the team's management of the case. Most team members will be primarily concerned with the physical management of the child. In the context of bonding and the development of communication it is essential that the psychological needs of the baby and the parents are recognised. Counselling should be directed to the exploration of the factors listed above, together with the provision of appropriate support. There is evidence that good communication development is more likely to take place within a well-adjusted family context. Time spent in counselling and support in the pre-speech period can be justified in cost-effective terms.

4 The clinician in the home locality has an important role to play in *preparing parents for appointments with team members*, for example through the preparation of questions to ask, reviewing these after the appointment and, where necessary, giving further explanations.

5 *Ensure that appropriate support is given for feeding difficulties.* In hospitals, except in undeveloped countries, there will be specialist staff available. This may include a speech clinician as well as specialist nurses and the orthodontist. Orthodontists may provide feeding plates and lip strapping where necessary. Back at home support may not be so readily available, so that the clinician and community nursing staff should work together.

In some countries there may be deeply entrenched views about feeding the baby in a supine position, and it may be difficult to convince parents of the importance of sitting the baby up to prevent choking and nasal regurgitation and to promote swallowing (**Sweeny**, 1989).

Teats with flaps to cover the cleft should only be used as a last resort. There are suggestions that poor feeding patterns may affect motor development and oro-sensory awareness. Some teats used, although improving feeding, may inhibit the usual tongue-thrusting pattern of suckling and may lead to reduced sensory awareness in the tongue-tip and alveolar ridge. **Morris & Klein** (1987) list five criteria for selecting a nipple. Clinicians should refer to this comprehensive work on pre-feeding skills which devotes a chapter to feeding cleft palate babies, while the leaflet by **Klein** (1988) is excellent for parents. Some culturally favoured foods such as curries and spices have been noted as causing more nasal regurgitation and may need to be avoided when the baby is going onto solids (**Sweeny**, 1989).

Just as important as the physical factors are the psychological implications for parents of having to spend hours feeding a hungry, distressed and sometimes exhausted baby, with the consequent increase in tension. This deprives mother and baby of the usually pleasurable opportunity in which early mother/baby bonding and interaction takes place. This may be of major consequence in relation to speech and language development. The unrepaired lip, even when concealed and brought together by strapping, may cause further distress to parents. In the developed world in most cases lip repairs will have been carried out by age three months. In some centres this is now done within a few days of birth.

6 *Parents need to be helped to maintain the stimulus for speech and language development.* Some parents will be anxious about their baby's ability to learn to speak and may unknowingly reduce their stimulus for speech and language both pre- and post-operatively. There is evidence that toddlers and children with cleft lip and/or palate are provided with fewer opportunities for speaking than their normal peers (**Spriestersbach**, 1973). This tendency needs to be counteracted. Parents should be told that there may be regression in vocalisations immediately after the operation to repair the palate (**Grunwell & Russell**, 1987). Special care needs to be taken to maintain language stimulus, even when a toddler is unintelligible. Attempts at speech should be positively rewarded and not corrected. Every opportunity should be taken for the input of normal models of language.

7 Current research shows that patterns of vocalisations in cleft palate babies differ in quality from those of their normal peers; therefore *the speech clinician should not only focus on counselling but also on specific intervention which lays down patterns of movement and sensory feedback on which speech sound development can be based* (*see below*).

8 *Parents should be shown how to stimulate babble patterns*, using the

range of placements within the vocal tract. Both assisted and imitated babble can be used.

9 *Provide demonstrations and guidelines for parents to carry out specific procedures directed towards the development of pre-speech motor skills.* These should include:

- ▶ Increasing sensory awareness;
- ▶ Increasing mobility and range of lip and tongue movements;
- ▶ Increasing the degree of mouth opening;

(*see further discussion below*). These procedures can be carried out both pre- and post-operatively. It is also important that they are maintained if palate repair is to be delayed. A number of ideas for working on oro-facial stimulation are provided by **Brookshire *et al*** (1980) and **Morris & Klein** (1987).

10 *Where assessment shows that speech sounds are not progressing to developmental norms, specific work should begin.* Of major importance is the development of plosives, which should appear around age 18 months. Clinicians will need to note variations in sound development in different languages.

11 *Parents should be fully involved in the assessment of their child's speech and language development.* This can be achieved at any age through ensuring that a parent is present at all stages of speech and language assessment and that they contribute data relevant to the evaluation process, by noting down or recording the child talking at home.

12 Children with cleft lip and/or palate have been found to be at risk in a wide range of developmental areas, such as social and cognitive development. *The speech clinician can provide a monitoring and screening role in all aspects of development and should liaise with health, social and educational services.*

13 *Monitor the way parents respond to and interact with their child. Ideally this should be done in the home setting to support observations made in the clinic.* The clinician in the specialist unit and the clinician in the home locality should liaise. Discussion with the health visitor will provide valuable information. Where indicated, help can be provided through the modelling of interactive behaviours. The dynamics of the family as a whole should be monitored, to assess whether it is helpful to the child's communication development.

14 *Ensure that other factors which may be detrimental to speech and language development receive appropriate management.* Children with cleft lip and palate are subject to the whole range of factors which may affect speech and language development in the rest of the population. This applies to phonological aspects as well as to other levels of language development. Take care not to focus solely on the identified physical condition, thereby overlooking other causative and maintaining factors.

15 *Note should be made of persisting indicators of inadequate velo-pharyngeal function post-operatively.* These would include marked hypernasality, nasal emission and grimace and lack of progress in the development of articulation skills. If these are observed, an opinion should be sought from the plastic surgeon. It should not be left until the child is nearing four years of age for a decision to be made about the adequacy of the velopharyngeal mechanism — children normally have an almost complete phonetic inventory by this age.

16 *If velopharyngeal closure is not adequate and further surgery is awaited it may still be possible to work on the sub-skills for speech:*

- ▶ Auditory;
- ▶ Sensory;
- ▶ Motor;
- ▶ Air-stream mechanisms;
- ▶ Articulatory placements.

Special attention should be paid to the treatment principle of not getting the child to do anything which results in excessive effort.

17 *Provide parents with an introduction to speech sound making.* They may need help in learning to recognise unwanted patterns such as glottal stops, nasal emission etc.

18 *Parents can be guided to carry out specific procedures on a daily basis with babies and toddlers.* The following areas should be worked on:

- ▶ Increase sensory awareness and movement (*Figure 7.1*);
- ▶ Encourage gentle air-stream through the mouth (*Figure 7.2*);
- ▶ Babble and sound making (*Figure 7.3*).

Further practical suggestions can be found in **Brookshire *et al*** (1980); **Morris & Klein** (1987) and **Wells** (1971).

BABIES		
Accepting oral stimulation		**Material**
Allow/encourage baby to play with soft (rubber) toys, suitable to put in mouth. This may get baby used to accepting objects into the mouth; may also help progress onto solid foods.		soft toys
Lips		
1	Stroking lips from top in midline encourages lip pursing.	
2	Gentle stimulation of lips with soft brush.	electric toothbrush
3	Rub lips with 'Vaseline', including upper lip scar. When lips are sticky, sensation of contact will be enhanced.	'Vaseline' or flavoured lip salve
4	Massage with facial sponge.	facial sponge
5	Make funny faces.	
6	Hold small object in mouth by lip pressure, while pulling to extract object.	button on string/ card
7	Paint face; special attention to lips.	face paints
8	Copy lip movement — encourage vocalisation, assisted babble etc.	

Mouth opening		
1	Copy wide-open mouth.	
2	Yawning.	
3	Encourage vocalisation with wide-open mouth.	
Tongue-tip around mouth and to alveolar ridge		
1	Increase sensory awareness in ridge and tongue-tip; stimulate with toothbrush. When teeth cleaning commences, this can be included.	ordinary or electric toothbrush
2	Press alveolar ridge hard with finger. Get child to place tongue-tip on pressed spot.	
3	Identify points with cotton swabs — can be used with water or juice. Use swabs which will not break if bitten.	swabs/juice
4	Use sticky substances to identify points.	jam
5	Ice/ice lolly for licking and stretching tongue-tip.	ice/ice lolly
6	Place food around outside of lips to encourage child to lick off.	
TODDLERS AND YOUNG CHILDREN		
If work is commenced at the toddler stage the above may be used as appropriate to establish base-line. The following activities are more suitable with more mature children. Where possible, and if child can co-operate, introduce mirror.		
1	Encourage inspection of own, parent's, clinician's mouth. Name parts appropriately.	
2	Imitate movements in mirror with parent/clinician.	
3	Imitate movements of doll with movable tongue.	
4	Oral movements accompanied by vowels, /ooooo/ /eeeee/, use exaggerated lip movement.	
5	Hold small object, flattened waxed straw, card etc between lips; gradually extend time of lip seal. Ensure object is not held by incisors. If lip seal cannot be maintained, establish short period of closure around small objects.	

Figure 7.1 ***Increasing sensory awareness and movement***

Working with Toddlers up to School Age

Many of the activities suggested in the figures can be used with toddlers and children up to school age. Activities can be extended and made more complex. However from about age three years it may be possible, if necessary, to work more directly on the development of articulatory skills. In all cases articulatory placement should be a priority, while manner can be

The aim of these activities is to establish the concept and sensation of air passing through the mouth. Activities will not improve an inadequate velopharyngeal mechanism. ALL ACTIVITIES SHOULD BE CARRIED OUT IN A GENTLE, RELAXED, EFFORTLESS WAY. DISCONTINUE IF TENSION OR NASAL GRIMACE IS NOTED. THE USE OF MUSICAL INSTRUMENTS IS NOT RECOMMENDED.	
1	Let child feel air-stream on back of hand.
2	Blowing activities to demonstrate result of air-stream: ▶ cotton wool; ▶ bubbles; ▶ feathers.
3	Blow cotton wool out of box (oral air-stream) while second piece of cotton wool on top of box (nasal air-stream) remains undisturbed.
4	Blowing into cupped hands, down tube etc (below nose) helps to establish the idea of where air should be passing.
5	Blowing down straw to move light objects on water (paper boats).
6	Imitate blowing up cheeks if child can achieve effortlessly. Let air burst out of mouth; paper bag bursting provides a model.
7	Introduce consonants, eg. /ffffffffff/ or /ssssssssss/ to be used in blowing; see result of oral air-stream by moving paper/candles.

Figure 7.2 ***Encouraging an oral air-stream***

worked on with those children where the velopharyngeal mechanism is competent or marginally competent.

Where the palate has not been repaired, alternative management, such as obturation, should begin to be considered by the team. Early obturation will not be easy because of difficulty in stabilising the appliance on primary dentition, and appliances will need to be changed frequently because of growth. In cases where palatal repair has taken place but the evidence is that velopharyngeal closure cannot be achieved, the team should discuss the need for, and timing of, further surgery. Continued speech intervention may be contraindicated, although language work should be maintained if necessary.

Parents will need support in coming to understand why further speech progress may not be possible until after surgery and why further work on speech is inadvisable. They should be counselled not to correct the child where improvement is not possible.

Speech or Language Intervention?

Measures to continue to encourage language development should always be maintained. If specific provision is being made to increase language skills, it is important that parents, play group leaders, nursery teachers and so on understand that these measures will not in fact improve speech skills.

There is some debate as to whether speech or language should be

1	Baby/toddler may be encouraged by feeling the vocalisations of clinician/parent.
2	Drumming fingers on lips to encourage labial sounds.
3	Assist child to produce contacts: bilabial, labio-dental, tongue up.
4	Imitation of oral versus nasal should be first distinction children are able to make.
5	Vegetative noises and spontaneous vocalisations should be imitated by parent/clinician to reinforce child and produce further vocalisations. UNDESIRABLE PATTERNS, eg. GLOTTALS, SHOULD NOT BE REINFORCED.
6	Hold baby/toddler close to face to watch CV combinations; include voiced/voiceless. Use variation of loudness and intonation.
7	General body activities of clapping/tapping help to introduce concepts of what has to be done in the oral cavity.
8	Repeated /wa/wa/wa/ with exaggerated lip rounding.
9	Encourage blowing (oral) interrupted by gentle stopping of air-stream by opening/closing lips or moving tongue up and down to alveolar ridge.
10	Feel larynx of parent/clinician to get idea of voice/voiceless, encourage child to feel own larynx in sound making.
11	Parents to stimulate sound making in pleasurable activities: feeding, bathing, playing.
12	Introduce play activities with specific associated vocalisations: bouncing ball, /b b b/; push; up etc. with associated actions.
13	Singing to /la/la/la/.

Figure 7.3 **Babbling and sound making**

worked on in those children where both are deficient. Ideally the two should be brought along together, so that, as language expands, improvements in speech ensure that the child has some chance of being understood. This then allows the adults (and older siblings) to expand and reinforce the child's talking. If parents do not appear to be instinctive language teachers, they should receive help through modelling and counselling. The help of staff in play groups and nursery schools should be enlisted.

Clinicians have a wide range of knowledge and skills in language development work which can be applied to the child with cleft palate. Attendance at a pre-school language group may be beneficial. Where language work is the identified aim, parents, teachers and clinicians will also be providing models for input for phonological development and correct realisation of target sounds. There is no harm in the adult repeating mispronounced words to provide a correct model, as long as this does not produce pressure or embarrassment and the child is not required to repeat.

Brookshire *et al* (1980) provide specific guidance on the development of language in young children with cleft palate.

Principles for Specific Work on Speech in Young Children

The procedures outlined in *Figures 7.1, 7.2* and *7.3* provide a good foundation for later speech work. The following principles should be considered:

1 Because of the subtleties of working on phonation and resonance, *direct work on resonance and phonation is not usually possible with most pre-school children.* Measures should be taken to discourage any obviously vocally abusive activities, such as those identified by **Wilson** (1987):

- Shouting, yelling and screaming;
- Loud and/or excessive talking;
- Loud whispering;
- Strained or explosive vocalisations;
- Abrupt glottal attack;
- Throat clearing;
- Reverse phonation;
- Coughing;
- Talking in noise.

Accepting that the vocal tract acts as a dynamic whole, it follows that, if articulation improves in association with less abuse of the mechanism, then the overflow effect of good adaptive movements will be to reduce resonatory and phonatory problems (*see also Chapter 8*).

2 Perceptual skills should be checked as a base-line to production. *The assessment of auditory skills should attend especially to recognition and discrimination.* Discriminatory work should be included up to the level of phonological contrast, through the use of play people, puppets and so on, named with minimal pairs. It is probably best to use nonsense words not locked into the child's repertoire. Where words are used, the *Best Ever* series of minimal pair pictures, which range from single sounds to voiceless/voiced final consonants and cluster contrasts, provides excellent pictorial material (**Taberham & Ball**, 1987).

3 *Auditory input should be closely tied to attempts at production.* The same nonsense words can be used as in the receptive tasks. This helps to avoid the trigger for learned articulatory patterns. Production is essential in laying down the patterns of movement and sensory awareness which need to become associated with target sounds. Excessive amounts of time should not be spent on auditory training, unless there is hearing impairment or assessment has shown inadequate auditory perceptual skills.

4 *Parents and other adults in contact with the child (teachers, grandparents etc) should be given careful explanations as to what should/or should not be corrected.* With the pre-school child this will be done in the context of increasing adults' understanding of the expected sequence of phonetic and phonological development. Remember to make a tape-recording of the discussions for the parent to take home.

5 *Correct articulation may be achieved even in the presence of persisting nasal emission.* In the presence of nasal emission or nasal snort it is sometimes difficult to analyse the exact place and manner of articulation. These may be found to be correct but overlaid and masked by the nasal emission. If place and manner are incorrect, they should be modified as far as possible. The establishment of place is of prime importance. It is also best to try to achieve a manner commensurate with normal phonetic/phonological development, even if the production remains weak and is masked to some extent by the nasal emission. See the examples in *Figure 7.4*.

	Target
/p^{F}/ is better than /ʔ/	/p/
/t͉^{F}/ is better than /ɦ/	/t/
/θ͉^{F}/ is better than /h/	/θ/

Figure 7.4 **Examples of sounds to aim for**

6 The point of entry into speech work is a subject of debate. Taking the position that phonological problems may stem from articulatory and phonetic ones due to physical limitations of production, *the point of entry for production at articulatory or phonetic levels is logical and acceptable.* Ideally CV production should be the start of the phonetic level. Imitation is the simplest way and should be attempted first. If this is not possible, the child should be taken back to the production of a single sound, as many sensory approaches as possible being used. (*See Figure 8.7 for ideas on sound elicitation.*)

7 In introducing new sounds the following factors should be considered:

- Developmental sequence;
- Level of difficulty, eg. in getting the air-stream to the front of the mouth;
- Ease in demonstrating, eg. most visible to least visible.

8 *Use any procedures which will show results*, eg.:

- Air-stream on back of hand;
- Feel larynx — voiced/voiceless;
- Show movement of air-stream — paper, feathers etc.

(*See Chapter 8.*)

9 *Gradually extend the phonetic repertoire to include sounds which are as near to the target as possible.* A decision will need to be made as to what is an acceptable realisation. Parents will need help with this and in accepting a half-way stage to correct production.

10 *A parent should always be present when working with pre-school children* as they are essential in carrying out the day-to-day practice. When possible it is valuable to tape-record the whole session, so that the parent can use this as a means of checking procedures of which they may feel unsure when they get home. A decision will need to be made on the advisability of the child hearing his own production.

The case example of Jeremy in *Chapter 10* illustrates the management of a pre-school child.

Chapter 8
Treatment Procedures for Speech

Treatment of Insufficient Nasality (Hyponasality) / *76*
Nose Blowing / *76*
Auditory Training and Production / *77*
Treatment of Excess Nasality (Hypernasal Resonance) / *77*
Treatment of Dysphonia / *79*
Treatment of Articulation / *81*
Treatment Principles for Articulatory and Phonetic Levels / *82*

CHAPTER 8
TREATMENT PROCEDURES FOR SPEECH

The treatment programme should be founded on a set of clearly stated aims and objectives, based on the assessment findings which give direction to the treatment plan. The plan will be made up of several components focused upon the remediation of identified needs. This kind of logical development is illustrated in Jeremy's case in *Chapter 10*. With many cleft palate individuals attention to the resonatory, phonatory, articulatory and phonetic aspects of speech will all be needed. These will now be considered separately, although in speech production they become integrated.

Treatment of Insufficient Nasality (Hyponasality)

(The range of resonatory qualities is illustrated in *Figure 2.1, page 17.*) If hyponasality is present it is most likely to be the result of insufficient nasal airway, caused by some form of nasal blockage, for example adenoidal growth, collapsed nostril/s, deflected septum, nasal polyps or a severe head cold. The physical cause of the problem should be established through ENT investigation, and medical or surgical intervention carried out where necessary. Hyponasality may sometimes occur after pharyngoplasty where the pharyngeal flap is too large and does not allow enough air into the nasal cavities. It may not be possible to change the resonance. However hyponasality is generally more socially acceptable than hypernasality.

As well as nasal blockage affecting nasality, the consonants /m/, /n/ and /ŋ/ will be denasalised. Inability to breathe through the mouth decreases the volume of air actually taken into the lungs, reducing the breath support for speech. Therefore there can be detrimental effects on the rate and intensity of speech. The identification of the cause of the hyponasality is the key to management. *Figure 8.1* illustrates management and treatment.

Nose Blowing

Many young children find it extremely difficult to learn to blow their nose and hyponasality may be present purely because the airway is not kept clear. Time should be spent in teaching nose blowing and establishing mouth breathing. First establish the idea of blowing out of the nose with closed lips. Get the child to puff down the nose to move a tissue or piece of cotton wool held on a shiny surface under the nose. Parents should be encouraged to do this with the child several times a day. Only when the concept of blowing down the nose has been established should the tissue/handkerchief be introduced. The child should be reminded to keep the lips sealed each time blowing into the handkerchief to remove mucus is attempted.

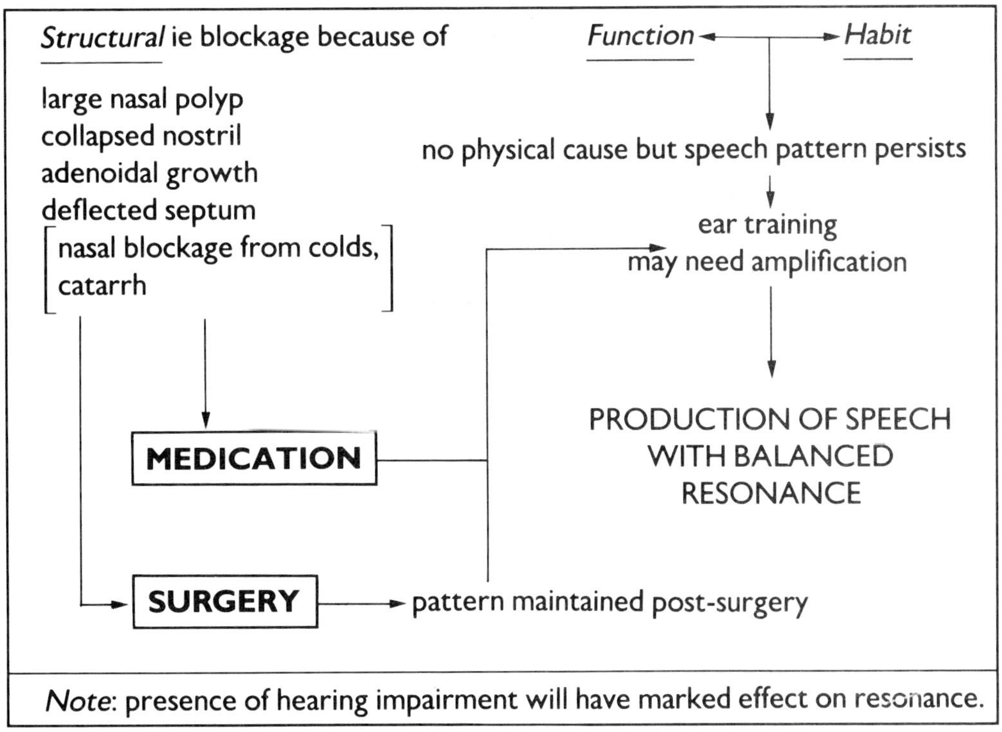

Figure 8.1 ***Management and treatment of hyponasality***

Auditory Training and Production

Resonatory patterns are learnt primarily through the auditory channel. The following procedures are suggested:

1 Ensure that the family models are not ones of hyponasality.

2 Carry out ear training, especially discrimination of balanced and hyponasal patterns.

3 Exercises in forward humming and moving onto vowels.

4 Exercises in producing clear contrasts between /m/ and /b/; /n/ and /d/.

5 Exercises in consonant contrasts of the above in words and sentences.

6 With an older child use reading passages with a preponderance of nasal consonants (see **Boone**, 1982 and **Fletcher**, 1972).

7 Use negative practice to contrast hypo- versus balanced resonance.

Frequent use of audio-recording should be made.

Treatment of Excess Nasality (Hypernasal Resonance)

This is a feature which frequently occurs in cleft palate cases. (Refer to *Chapter 2, page 16* for the factors leading to hypernasality. These must all be considered in the treatment plan.) Nasal emission and nasal grimace will frequently be found in cases where excess nasality is present. *Figure 8.2* summarises approaches to management and treatment. Note the importance of establishing the status of the velopharyngeal mechanism. Occasionally hypernasality is the only deviant speech feature and it is a difficult feature to treat in isolation; careful analysis of all the possible contributory

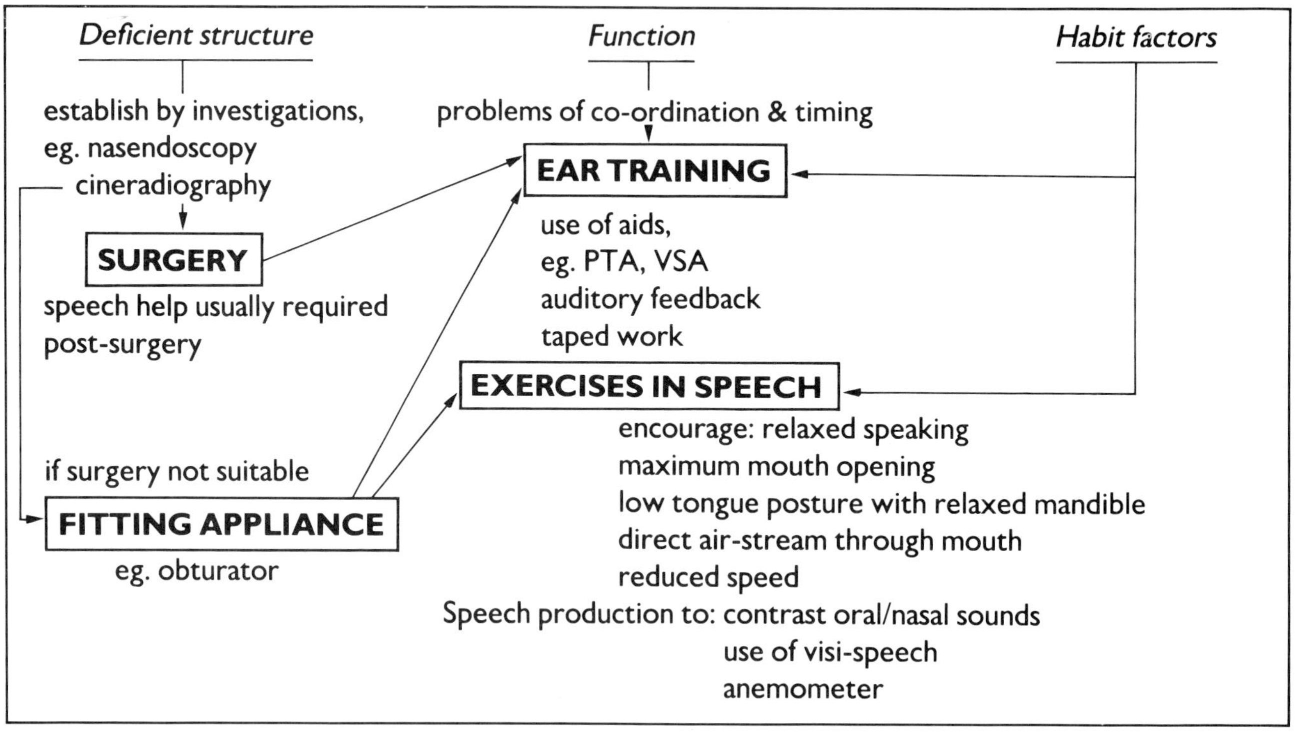

Figure 8.2 ***Management and treatment of hypernasality***

factors should be made and procedures adopted for their modification. Generally other speech parameters, especially articulation, will require treatment. Work on all areas will need to be integrated.

The treatment of hypernasality is directed to changing resonance and does not affect velopharyngeal closure. If the latter is inadequate, ideally it should first be surgically managed. In some cases surgery may not be possible. Hypernasality may be reduced by using the following approaches:

1. Ensure that there is adequate breath support for speech. If not, work on breathing exercises and breath control.
2. Establish that the patient understands the nature of the feature being worked on, by using imitation and recorded examples, as well as understanding the mechanisms by which the excess nasality is caused.
3. Ear training may be necessary to recognise both undesired and desired target quality.
4. Encourage low tongue carriage.
5. Encourage adequate mouth opening. Restricted mouth opening and high tongue carriage often go together. Reducing speed may enable greater oral openness. Use a mirror when comparing patient and clinician. Increase insight into mouth opening in speech through observation of others, such as family, friends, or people on television. Use **Boone**'s (1982) self-practice sheets facilitating approach — 'Open Mouth' — with older patients. This is used in the case of Mr N, outlined in *Chapter 10*.
6. If the patient finds mouth opening difficult, general relaxation may help. Pay particular attention to posture. In some instances (eg. Klippel Feil syndrome) mouth opening may be anatomically restricted. Establish the head posture which facilitates maximum opening.
7. Establish an adequate degree of loudness. Many cleft palate individuals speak at a reduced volume. This may be because the air source cannot be used efficiently. Reduced loudness exacerbates problems of intelligi-

bility. Improvement in this area may have significance for communicative effectiveness as a whole. Reduced loudness will also be found where mouth opening is restricted. Increase in loudness and mouth opening should be worked on concurrently.

8 Explore concepts to help the patient grasp what is meant by oral air-stream, for example by pulling objects out of the mouth like a magician — string, scarves or a long string of spaghetti.

9 Identify and establish optimum pitch. Some speakers adopt an inappropriately high pitch, thus increasing the perception of nasality.

10 Take care not to precipitate laryngeal elevation in the attempt to reduce hypernasality, as this will lead to vocal hyperfunction and dysphonia.

11 Audio-record examples of the individual's improved resonance and play back as a base-line for generalised production.

12 Practise CV sequences/words in which desired resonance can be most easily maintained.

13 Use anemometry to provide immediate feedback on the amount of nasal air-flow.

14 Practise sequences of speech which are low in nasals to help maintain the target resonance.

15 Where it is established that, although velopharyngeal closure can be achieved, there are difficulties in the synchrony, weakness and timing of movements, consider the use of a palatal training appliance and visual speech aid, with cases of suitable age (*see Chapter 9*).

Treatment of Dysphonia

Point 10 above again emphasises the close relationship between resonance and phonation. Treatment of the phonatory level must therefore be linked with treatment of other speech features. Abusive activities associated with maladaptive articulation, especially the constant use of the glottis as an articulator, may lead to laryngeal and phonatory changes. It follows that improvements in articulation are likely to lead to less vocal abuse and improved phonation.

When a child uses reduced volume in an attempt to hide speech problems, especially those of hypernasality and nasal emission, a weak breathy voice quality results. In non-cleft palate children most dysphonias are associated with vocally abusive activities, such as excessive yelling, making strange loud vocal noises in play, throat clearing and coughing (*see Chapter 7*). These behaviours should be identified and managed in the child with cleft palate, so that vocal hyperfunction is not presumed to be purely related to tension in talking associated with an inadequate velopharyngeal mechanism. Make note of vocal behaviour in other family members, especially siblings.

When dysphonia has been identified, refer to the ENT specialist for investigation of the status of the larynx. Where nodules are found in young children surgical removal is not usually advised. Vocally abusive behaviours should be identified and managed in therapy. This will require the close co-operation of parents and school. *Figure 8.3* summarises general approaches to the management and treatment of dysphonia, while *Figures 8.4* and *8.5* provide suggestions for treatment. Readers are also directed to **Boone** (1982); **Fawcus** (1986); **Martin** (1988) and **Wilson** (1987).

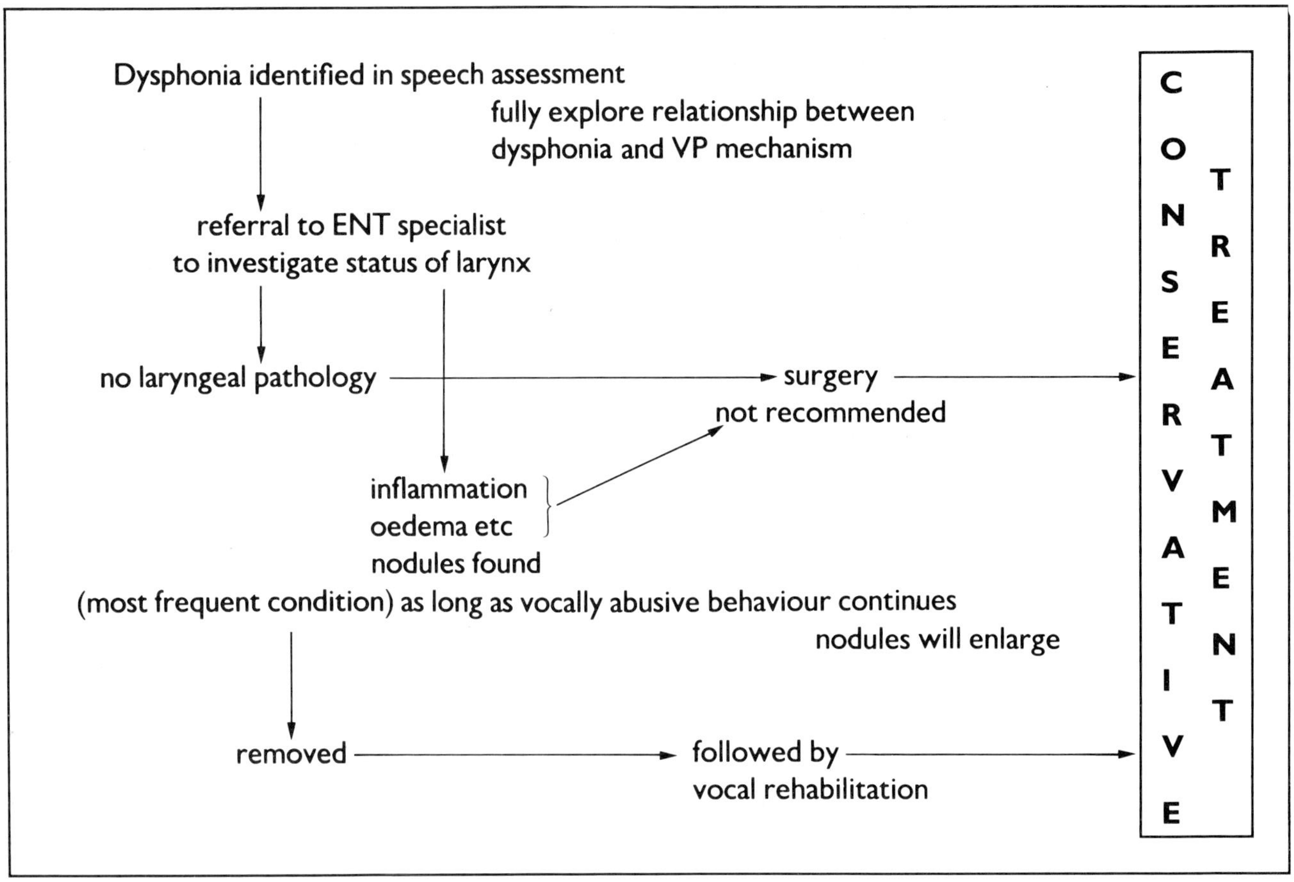

Figure 8.3 ***Management and treatment of dysphonia***

1	Help client to understand how voice is produced.
2	Understand the harmful behaviours.
3	Older children and adults should keep a diary recording vocally abusive behaviour.
4	Consider the need for environmental monitoring, eg. reducing noise in home which the child has to speak over. With adults consider the work situation.
5	Monitoring of all vocally abusive behaviours, eg. yelling, shouting, screaming, making funny vocal noises in play, throat clearing. Both school and home may need to be involved in monitoring.
6	Relaxation to reduce effort in speaking; gently phonate when relaxed. Pay particular attention to posture.
7	Practise gentle approach to talking; pay particular attention to vowels; /h/ can be used as a way into vowels but care should be taken not to precipitate breathy quality.
8	Use visi-speech to identify hard/soft attack. Hard attack is not the same as the use of glottals for the articulation of some sounds, although the two may frequently go together.
9	Auditory discrimination to identify hard attack in others and self.
10	Use of improved phonation in various practice and role-play contexts.

Figure 8.4 ***The treatment of vocal hyperfunction***

1	Help client to understand how voice is produced.
2	Attend to posture.
3	Auditory discrimination to identify optimal level in self and others.
4	Presence of hearing loss needs to be taken into account.
5	Masking may be used to increase volume.
6	Try pitch changes to establish where volume is easiest.
7	If monotone has been identified as part of the soft voice pattern, work on increasing the pitch range (**McWilliams *et al*** 1984).
8	Talking to someone at a distance to increase volume without tension.
9	The 'pushing' approach should be used with caution, in case it precipitates hard attack. (In the 'pushing' technique, the chest is fixed, eg. by pushing away from a surface, such as a wall, to produce phonation — /a/ — effortful sound.)
10	Use amplified voice to get individual used to hearing a louder voice.
11	Provide opportunities in clinic and environment to speak out.

Note: Care needs to be taken not to produce hyperfunction. Treatment should be stopped if hypernasality increases. Any tendency to produce/increase a nasal grimace should be monitored. Some individuals, when encouraged to speak more loudly, may not be able to do so because of energy loss through the velopharyngeal mechanism.

Figure 8.5 ***The treatment of vocal hypofunction***

In some children and adults where vocally abusive behaviour is firmly established because of compensation for an inadequate velopharyngeal mechanism, it may not be possible to change the vocal behaviour until a better mechanism is provided through surgery. This applies both to cases of cleft palate and to cases of congenital velopharyngeal incompetence. The clinician should press for surgical intervention as soon as possible.

Voice therapy should normally be carried out on a trial basis, information on the status of the larynx having been sought through the ENT specialist. If treatment of dysphonia increases the excess nasality, direct attention to the voice should cease, except if treatment is designed to reduce vocal nodules.

Treatment of Articulation

A comprehensive and excellent review of the treatment of articulation disorders in cleft palate can be found in **McWilliams *et al*** (1984). There is some research evidence that speech therapy improves the articulation of cases with velopharyngeal competence and borderline velopharyngeal competence, and, although this evidence is still rather scant, it is probably sufficient to give clinicians confidence to undertake treatment in this area. **Albery** (1989) believes that the treatment of articulation is the area in which the clinician can make the largest contribution to the improvement of speech. Clinical experience supports this view. It must be recognised, however, that speech therapy does not in itself improve velopharyngeal closure and where closure is in question discussion on the need for further surgery should be maintained with the plastic surgeon.

The point of entry to improve speech at phonetic and phonological levels may be through:

1 Enhancement of motor skills;
2 Improvement of articulatory skills;
3 Direct work on target sound or feature;
4 Work on phonemic contrasts.

Usually all these areas will need some attention. Approaches to the enhancement of motor skills were discussed, in relation to young children, in the previous chapter. The same principles of achieving awareness, sensitivity and mobility of structures can be applied to all age groups. Procedures such as those used in proprioceptive neuromuscular facilitation (PNF) may be found beneficial.

The following section will focus mainly on the improvement of articulation and the production of target sounds, but will refer to improvement of motor skills as a base for these as well as referring forward to working on phonemic contrasts essential for phonological development.

Treatment Principles for Articulatory and Phonetic Levels

The following principles should be considered in approaching the management of speech at the articulatory and phonetic levels:

1 Take into consideration all relevant psychological and social factors. For example, the older child needs to be motivated about self-change, while the adolescent may be much more concerned about appearance than speech. If a child is over-conscious about speech and coping with a new situation, for example starting a new school, it might be advisable to delay the start of treatment.

2 Make sure the child/adult and all those concerned, eg. parents and professionals, understand the nature of the speech difficulties and the likely outcomes of the speech intervention.

3 Articulation must first have been carefully analysed, using a fine phonetic transcription. Speech patterns need to be examined in all phonetic contexts as this might provide important points of entry for change.

4 Help all involved to achieve insight about speech production through explanation and demonstration. With children the *Tongue Position Charts* (**Frey**, 1987) may be used. Add information on voicing and the position of the soft palate.

5 Establish why the articulatory/phonetic difficulties persist; that is, do they relate to:

- Hearing impairment;
- Inadequate velopharyngeal competence;

- Malocclusion;
- Poor sensory awareness etc.

6 Ensure that all has been done or is going to be done to remediate/alleviate any of the above factors.

7 Establish the ability to carry out the prerequisite motor and articulatory skills.

8 Ensure everyone involved understands the implications of various management procedures on speech, for example that the patient having a pharyngoplasty will not come out of hospital with normal speech, nor will orthodontic treatment bring about dramatic speech change.

9 Establish the aims of intervention; for example, normal speech or perhaps only improved articulation, with increased intelligibility. (Improvement may be constrained by persisting malocclusion, intellectual factors, borderline velopharyngeal competence etc.) Consider the controversy, already outlined, as to whether articulation should or should not precede pharyngoplasty. **Albery** (1989) suggests a flexible approach to this dilemma. The decision should be based on age, severity of the speech problem, possible timing of surgery and the views of the surgeon. Often a period of diagnostic therapy should be undertaken. This will help to establish whether or not surgery is necessary. The ability to produce plosives and fricatives will be an important indicator.

10 Where necessary, work on auditory receptive skills prior to or concurrent with production. Training should establish the relationship between perception and production for self-monitoring. (Note the controversy over perception and production, for further discussion of which see **Elbert & Gierut**, 1986.)

11 Where possible, follow the normal pattern of phonetic and phonological development.

12 From stimulability tests and the client's level of awareness, decide where to start. A client may sometimes be concerned about a sound which is not of great consequence functionally. Discuss such factors. If it is a sound which is likely to be corrected easily it could be a good starting point for progress and motivation.

13 Use as many sensory channels as possible, including the fitting of an acrylic dental plate with target ridges (see **Stuffins**, 1989), or a plate with an exposed alveolar ridge to establish alveolar placement. Use an auditory trainer for children with hearing impairment.

14 With older children and adults the use of electropalatography (EPG) can make a major breakthrough in achieving articulatory change where patterns have been deeply entrenched (*see Chapter 9* and **Hardcastle *et al***, 1989).

15 Start direct work on articulation as early as possible (this will have been preceded by the kind of programme outlined in *Chapter 7*). The elimination of glottal articulation as early as possible is of major importance. **Albery** (1989) recommends the use of direct speech work with children as young as three years.

16 *Always encourage a gentle approach to articulation production.* This will discourage glottalisation and nasal grimace. If audible nasal emission is present, any increase in tension will exacerbate the nasal turbulence.

17 Where a new sound can only be produced in isolation, contrast with sounds which are easily articulated to introduce the idea that sounds are in sequences; eg. /f ⟶ /l//f ⟶ /l/. At this stage the exercises need not be within the phonotactic possibilities of a language. Sometimes the patient will find it easier to produce C + C rather than C + V combinations.

18 Use articulatory drills to establish articulatory ease. After single sounds can be produced with ease, *move to larger units as quickly as possible.* Use of a known context should be avoided initially, as these are likely to trigger established articulatory patterns.

19 In cases of unrepaired cleft palate, work on articulation should be carried out. Articulatory placement should be the main goal. Ensure that there is not too much stress placed on a child. Short periods of spaced intervention should be adopted. An obturator with articulatory ridges may be beneficial.

20 The practice of closing the nares to achieve oral air-stream in the production of a sound should be used sparingly: it is controversial, as it could possibly overcome the necessity to achieve velopharyngeal closure. It may be used in the initial stage of eliciting a new sound, and in establishing feedback.

21 In some instances therapy may need to be suspended for surgical or dental treatment.

22 Help the client and others to understand what is an acceptable production of a particular sound. For example, /f/ may still be accompanied by audible nasal emission, but placement must be labio-dental, with some air passing through this contact to create friction, even if this is weak.

23 While one sound is being worked on in connected speech, other sounds can be introduced, so that various sounds or features will be worked on concurrently at different levels. This can include some sounds at the phonological level where the sound can be produced with ease or in a way that has been identified as acceptable. A chart can be used to remind everyone involved where they should be working. A proforma is shown in *Figure 8.6* (this may be copied for school and home use).

24 Explore patient/parent expectations: help all involved to understand what to expect, for example that there is a long way to go between an individual being able to produce a new sound in isolation, in CV combinations or even in single words, and spontaneous use in connected speech. Parents, grandparents, teachers and others involved should be discouraged from over-correcting or expecting too much too soon. Family and school counselling should be undertaken.

25 Constantly lead the individual towards evaluating their own speech standard. With older children and adults, self-monitoring should be a first priority in treatment.

26 Consider the relationship of speech work at the articulatory and phonetic level to phonology. The principles which may be applied in phonological therapy may not always be applicable to children with articulatory difficulties. The principle that 'teaching one member of a cognate pair will facilitate the accurate production of the other sound in that pair' (**Elbert & Gierut**, 1986) may not apply. For example, that teaching /z/ will lead to improvement in the production of /s/ may not happen in cleft palate cases because the physical apparatus limits the

SOUND	SHOULD BE USED SPONTANEOUSLY MAY NEED OCCASIONAL REMINDING	IN PRACTICE WORDS IN ALL POSITIONS SPONTANEOUS IN SOME WORDS	IN ISOLATION AND EXERCISES	CAN'T MANAGE YET DON'T CORRECT

Figure 8.6 ***Where we are with sounds***

child's ability to produce /s/, although /s/ /z/ contrasts are within the child's phonological competence.

27 Phonemic contrasts should be built into the therapy programme. The goal of articulation therapy is to enable the child to use an expanded or complete phonetic inventory in the phonological system. Opportunities should be provided for the child to try out new-found skills to see if they work.

28 Where secondary surgery has been carried out to improve the velopharyngeal mechanism, a year should be allowed for the new mechanism to become fully established (**McWilliams *et al***, 1984). If treatment has been satisfactory in terms of frequency of attendance and provision, co-operation, application, family support and appropriateness of treatment, and still there is little or no improvement, or articulation improves but nasal emission persists, refer back to the plastic surgeon.

The whole area of phonological therapy will not be considered further in this volume as it is dealt with amply elsewhere (see **Ingram**, 1976; **Grunwell**, 1982; **Elbert & Gierut**, 1986 and **Lancaster & Pope**, 1989). The same principles can usually be applied to the cleft palate child, as long as the physical limitations are taken fully into account.

The first job for the clinician, and sometimes one which is difficult to achieve, is to elicit the target sound as well as to eliminate any unwanted pattern. *Figures 8.7, 8.8* and *8.9* provide suggestions for sound elicitation. Further suggestions can be found in **Albery** (1989); **Morley** (1970) and **Wells** (1971). The figures have been developed from some of the suggestions by these authors, as well as from techniques used and found valuable in the author's clinical experience.

GENERAL: ELICITING PLOSIVES

Only plosives, fricatives (*Figure 8.8*) and affricates (*Figure 8.9*) are being included, as these are the sounds which present the greatest difficulty for individuals with cleft palate. English sounds only have been included. The principles of manner can easily be transferred to other sounds requiring the same manner. Increasing sensory awareness of place and heightening the auditory awareness of fine differences in place should be facilitated.

PRINCIPLES

Carry out auditory work first, and continue this along with work on production. Always try imitation first; if this fails use a mirror next. Some children find this confusing and distracting. Consider the dimensions of both place and manner. Use diagrams whenever possible.

Note: Do not introduce plosives unless nasals in same place have been established; eg. do not introduce /p/b/ unless /m/ is present. Firm, but not tense, contacts should be the goal.

Bilabial plosives: /p/b/

ACHIEVING MANNER & VOICING	ACHIEVING PLACE
1 Use terms to help develop appropriate concepts, eg. plosives: short sounds, bursts, puffs of air; voiceless: puffy sounds; voiced: buzzy sounds. 2 Start with voiceless. Interrupt gentle air-stream. Show visible result of puff of air-stream. 3 Strengthen lips for plosion by maintaining seal against resistance. Puff out cheeks before release. 4 Feel larynx for /b/. Take care to avoid the glottal in the voiced. Discourage over-effort, which will precipitate glottal.	1 Develop general awareness of articulators by increasing sensory awareness. Get patient to identify place used for plosives by clinician/parent. 2 Good lip movement in /w/ is prerequisite. 3 Rub lips with 'Vaseline' to facilitate contact. 4 Imitate silent open/closing of lips, gradually introduce gentle breath. 5 Hum with pressed lips, followed by /p/ or /b/; helps to establish placement. 6 Test stimulability in all phonotactic positions, to find easiest context. 7 Imitate silently words which include bilabial plosives; especially useful to focus on place and introduce voiceless.

Alveolar plosives: /t/d/

Note: Frequently replaced by glottal. Lacks precise tongue-tip contact. May be accompanied by nasal emission.

ACHIEVING MANNER & VOICING

1. Nature of sounds: short/burst/puff.
2. Sound concepts: tapping /t/t/t/; knocking /d/d/d/
3. Voiceless first.
4. Use symbols for voiced.
5. Use diagrams to show voicing.
6. Feel larynx for /d/.

ACHIEVING PLACE

1. Children stories about tongue activities; eg. 'Mr Tongue'.
2. Adolescents/adults use articulatory diagrams.
3. Head forward to facilitate place. Clinician press hard on 'spot'* on alveolar ridge; patient press 'spot'.
4. Lift tongue to 'spot' — use mirror.
5. Place small dental elastic between tongue-tip and 'spot' — hold, carry out of mouth on tongue-tip, return to 'spot', still holding elastic.
6. Use /n/ as place for start.
7. Increase sensory awareness in tongue-tip; brushing etc. Practise pointing tongue-tip.
8. Use EPG if appropriate age etc.

*'spot' place of contact; tongue-tip to alveolar ridge: see **Barrett & Hanson** (1978).

Velar Plosives: /k/g/

Note: May be replaced by glottal plosive or fricative. Sometimes achieving the exact place of contact is difficult in cases of cleft of soft palate. Will need auditory work to distinguish: /k/g/ (velar) from /ç/j/(palatal), and /q/G/ (uvular).

ACHIEVING MANNER & VOICING

1. Concepts: gun; tapping; knocking.
2. Care to be taken in introducing /g/ gently, because closeness of articulation contact to larynx may trigger glottal.
3. Use diagrams to show different parts of vocal tract and functions: tongue and velum tap for plosives. Vocal cords buzz.

ACHIEVING PLACE

1. Use mirror and diagrams.
2. Concepts for tongue working at back of mouth — clinician touch place with spatula, patient with finger.
3. Use big open mouth.
4. Tap under chin at base of tongue to identify place and encourage movement.
5. Introduce /k/ and /g/ next to high vowel: encourages high back tongue movement; high back tongue movement: /i:k/and /i:g/. May find easier in VCV, eg. /ɪkɪ/ /ɪgɪ/.

Figure 8.7 ***Eliciting new sounds: plosives***

GENERAL: ELICITING FRICATIVES

Use terms to help the development of appropriate concepts for production; long, gentle, quiet for voiceless. Continually guard against tendencies to try too hard and precipitate nasal grimace.

Labio-dental: /f/v/

Note: Place may be used but lacks friction through mouth, or may be accompanied by nasal emission. May be absent or replaced by glottal or pharyngeal fricative. Labio-dental usually easiest fricative to achieve first as it develops early and is easily visible.

ACHIEVING MANNER & VOICING	ACHIEVING PLACE
1 Establish gentle air-stream through mouth without stricture. 2 Feel air-stream from parent/ clinician. 3 Feel voice/no voice at larynx. 4 Production of VC first may be easiest, as allows sound to be held on and avoids triggering of old pattern which intrudes when moving from vowel to consonant.	1 Use mirror. 2 Manually assist patient to achieve labio-dental contact. 3 Increase awareness of contact point on lower lip: touching/rubbing. 4 Prolong friction initially to increase sensory and auditory awareness. 5 If incisors are missing, use of the upper gum ridge to lower lip will produce an auditorially acceptable sound.

ENCOURAGE SOFT CONTACT TO ALLOW EFFECTIVE FRICTION FROM GENTLE AIR-STREAM.

Alveolar fricatives: /s/z/

Usually found the most difficult fricative to achieve; requires high level of intra-oral air pressure and precise articulatory movements.

ACHIEVING MANNER & VOICING	ACHIEVING PLACE
1 Feel air-stream from clinician/parent on hand. 2 Concepts of fine air-stream: eg. single thread out of mouth as opposed to several threads for /f/.	1 Press 'spot' — to identify place. 2 Lift tongue-tip up to 'spot' stimulated by pressing on alveolar ridge. 3 Exercises to strengthen tongue-tip. 4 Experiment to see if patient finds easiest to produce with lowered or raised tongue-tip; tip needs to be strengthened, whether used in lowered or raised position. 5 Tongue-tip with elastic exercise.

	6 Establish lip spread with teeth close together, but not clenched. 7 May be facilitated by using /s/z/ next to /t/d/; eg. hats, buds, etc, or cut some; out soon; loud zoo etc.
Palato-alveolar: /ʃ/ʒ/	
ACHIEVING MANNER & VOICING	**ACHIEVING PLACE**
1 Use terms to help concepts of 'thick' stream of air as opposed to thin stream for /s/z/.	1 Awareness of broad palatal contact, with sides of tongue pressing up to side teeth. 2 Forward squared lips — mirror use. 3 Use EPG to show place.

Figure 8.8 **Eliciting new sounds: fricatives**

GENERAL: ELICITING AFFRICATES	
Affricates: /tʃ/dʒ/	
Usually leave until last because they are normally last in developmental sequence. Probably best to leave until /t/d/ and /ʃ/ʒ/ can be produced.	
ACHIEVING MANNER & VOICING	**ACHIEVING PLACE**
1 Explore appropriate concepts; eg. sneeze for /tʃ/. 2 Auditory work to compare fricatives/affricates. 3 Slow take away. 4 May find easiest in contrastive pair; eg. eat vs each; pat vs patch; led vs ledge; wed vs wedge. 5 Best not to use words in child's vocabulary which trigger old patterns. With older children/adults, use nonsense words.	1 May be elicited from place of plosive element, ie /t/ > /tʃ/; /d/ > /dʒ/. 2 Place for /t/d/ with slow release. Use of EPG where appropriate.

Figure 8.9 **Eliciting new sounds: affricates**

CHAPTER 9
INTRODUCTION TO INSTRUMENTATION

Nasal Anemometry/*92*
What is it?/*92*
The Hardware/*92*
Use of Nasal Anemometry/*93*
Palatal Training Appliance (PTA)/*94*
Indications for Use/*94*
What is it?/*94*
Suitable Patients/*95*
Speech Intervention Alongside Appliance Wearing/*95*
Visual Speech Aid (VSA)/*95*
Introducing the VSA/*95*
Design Modification/*96*
Evaluation of Progress/*96*
Cost-effectiveness/*97*
Electropalatography (EPG)/*97*
The Equipment/*98*
Use in Treatment/*99*
Suitable Cases/*99*
Availability/*99*
Nasendoscopy/*100*
Suppliers of Equipment/*100*
Electropalatography/*100*
Nasal Anemometer, PTA and VSA/*100*
Micronose/*100*

CHAPTER 9
INTRODUCTION TO INSTRUMENTATION

This chapter is designed to serve as a quick guide to the appliances generally available, indicating their usefulness. Full accounts on design of the instruments are available elsewhere. If the reader decides that one of the instrumental procedures might be of use to a particular client they should consult the appropriate reference sources before proceeding further.

Nasal Anemometry

What is it?

Anemometry is the measurement of wind force. Nasal anemometry has been designed to measure the force of air passing through the nose during speech. It was developed and described for clinical use by **Ellis *et al*** (1978). **Huskie** (1989) gives a full account of its use as an assessment and diagnostic tool, while **Stuffins** (1989) considers its use in treatment.

The Hardware

The part of the equipment to be used in clinic is portable and relatively inexpensive. It consists of:

- ▶ A stereo recorder;
- ▶ A sensing head with nasal mask;
- ▶ A control unit;
- ▶ A microphone.

This equipment is used to record the client's speech and nasal air-flow. The cassette recording made is sent to a centre for analysis and the provision of a print-out (in England to Exeter University) as illustrated in *Figure 9.1*. The speech sample recorded usually consists of 10 stimulus words with a range of sounds including high-pressure consonants.

The sensing head (thermistor), which is used to measure the air-flow, is mounted in a rubber anaesthetic mask for older children and adults, while a smaller acrylic mask can be used with younger children. The control box houses a meter which indicates the amount of air-flow at the time of recording. This can therefore be used for monitoring by the clinician and patient at the time of speaking, and so can serve as a treatment tool. A special 'training model' is available for use purely in providing feedback; with this no recording is made, but air-flow is indicated on the meter. It is reported to be over-sensitive to environmental air changes (**Stuffins**, 1989).

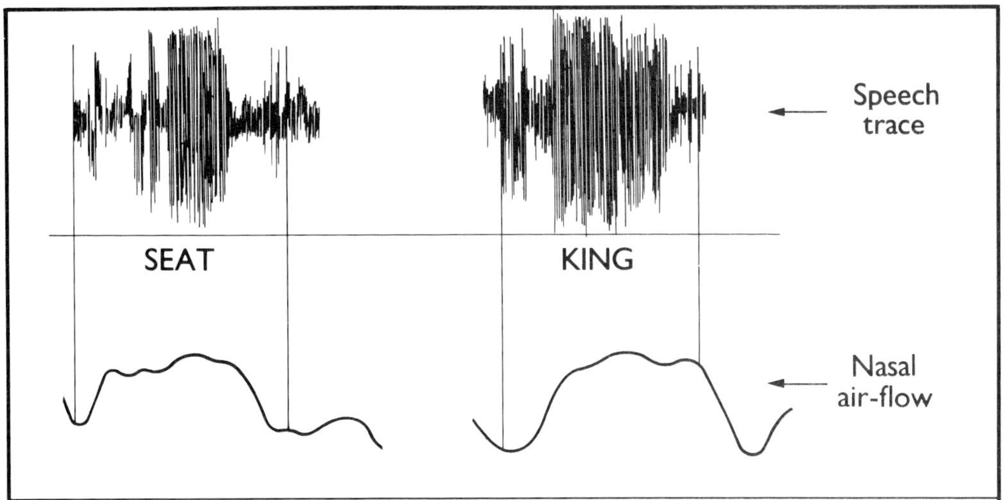

Note: Excess nasal air-flow.

Figure 9.1 ***Anemometry print-out of excess nasal air-flow in speaker with velopharyngeal incompetence***

Use of Nasal Anemometry

1 As an objective measurement of nasal air-flow, for recording and comparison.

2 As a treatment instrument to provide feedback.

3 Analysis of the recording provides information on:
   (a) the presence of excessive air-flow in consonant production where nasal air-flow is not normally present;
   (b) the points at which nasal air-flow occurs, ie whether it is purely on pressure consonants, persists across the speech pattern including vowels, or is most marked next to nasal consonants.

4 Recordings can be taken over time and compared in order to evaluate the efficacy of speech treatment or the outcomes of operative procedures.

5 Can be used in cases with oro-nasal fistula by taking recordings with fistula open or closed with an obturator or dental wax. This will help to identify whether the air escape is through the fistula or through the velopharyngeal mechanism.

Advantages

1 Generally available and not too expensive to have for departmental clinical equipment.

2 The procedure is only mildly invasive: the client needs to accept wearing the face mask.

3 It provides the most objective measure of nasal air-flow easily available to clinicians.

Disadvantages

1 Wearing the mask sometimes leads to changes in respiration and alterations in resonatory qualities. If the rubber mask is too tight or not correctly positioned nasal air-flow may be impeded.

2 No information is provided on the overall quality of speech, only on the amount of air-flow.

3 The recording has to be sent away for analysis, therefore results are not immediate.

Palatal Training Appliance (PTA)

The palatal training appliance used most frequently in the UK today was described by **Tudor & Selley** in 1974. They designed the appliance to produce 'some lifting of the soft palate'. However they found that it also acted as a training appliance. The clinical use has been described by **Curle** (1979); **Selley** (1979) and **Stuffins** (1989).

Indications for Use

The PTA might be prescribed for a patient who has a soft palate of sufficient length to reach the pharyngeal wall to achieve closure, but with muscular weakness and/or inco-ordination leading to velopharyngeal incompetence and consequent speech symptomotology. The speech clinician needs to work closely with the dental specialist for the fitting and monitoring of the use of the appliance.

What is it?

The construction is described by **Selley** (1979). An acrylic plate which carries the loop of stainless steel wire (*see Figure 9.2*) is made from impressions of the patient's palate. The wire should be adjusted so that it only just touches the soft palate where palatal lift would normally be expected. The loop should not put any pressure on the palate. Providing oral hygiene is good, the plate can be worn night and day, including when eating. The speech clinician can play an important role in helping patients to maintain good oral hygiene.

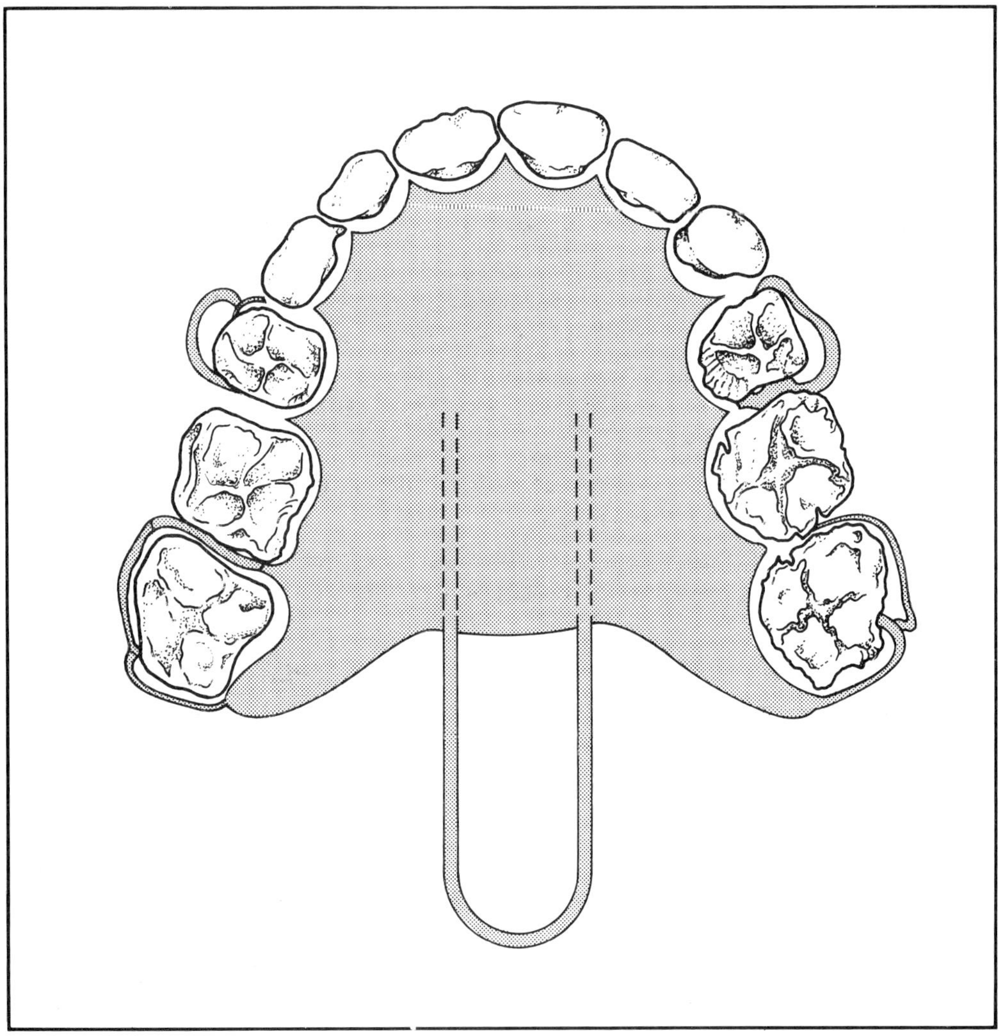

Figure 9.2 ***Palatal training appliance***

Suitable Patients

This appliance can be used with a wide age range of patients, providing the impressions can be taken and the appliance retained. **Stuffins** (1989) reports the use of a PTA with a child of three and a half years. PTAs tend to be prescribed for individuals who have already had a considerable amount of speech help. This may make continued treatment, even with the fitting of the appliance, an uphill task. While the appliance is being made it may be beneficial to suspend treatment. This will stabilise the speech standard to be used as a base-line against which change can be measured. It also gives the patient a break from intervention before work starts again on an intensive basis, as soon as the appliance is fitted.

The use of the PTA is also prescribed for drooling, swallowing problems, nasal regurgitation and some dysarthrias, where the inadequate function of the velopharyngeal mechanism is central in the speech breakdown.

Speech Intervention Alongside Appliance Wearing

Ideally the selection of the PTA as a treatment method should be made as early as possible. This can only be achieved through careful evaluation of the speech mechanism and an analysis of the speech. When the appliance is fitted, speech intervention should commence so that the potential for any improvement can be maximised.

The appliance may need to be worn for a year, although **Stuffins** (1989) described cases of the plate being worn for up to three and a half years. Some individuals may find it difficult to go without the plate and a gradual period of withdrawal may be needed. When the plate is withdrawn, audio-recording of maintained improvement will help to reassure the individual that speech has not regressed.

Visual Speech Aid (VSA)

The PTA with speech intervention may be sufficient to bring about speech improvement in some individuals. However, where the co-ordination of speech and the soft palate is a major problem, the addition of visual feedback to the system can be of benefit. This requires the making of a second plate in which the simple wire loop is replaced by two electrodes (*see Figure 9.3*). The electrodes are connected by insulated wire to a six-volt control box, which houses a small light. When the VSA is worn the soft palate rests on the electrodes. When the circuit is completed by soft palate contact the light in the control box goes on. When the circuit is broken by raising the soft palate the light is extinguished. In this way the patient receives feedback on the position of the soft palate. The VSA is used for practice periods only; these should be carried out several times a day. The clinician must ensure that the patient is able to work alone or under appropriate supervision. With some children this may sometimes be carried out more regularly in school. The control box will need to be available for practice.

Introducing the VSA

The VSA should be introduced only when an individual is used to wearing the PTA. A period of three weeks is usually recommended (**Selley**, 1979). When the VSA is introduced into treatment the PTA should still be worn at all other times as recommended by the dental specialist and clinician. Leaving the plate out at night may be important for oral hygiene. Some patients complain that they feel a 'hot fizzy' sensation from the electrodes; this needs frequent monitoring and adjustment.

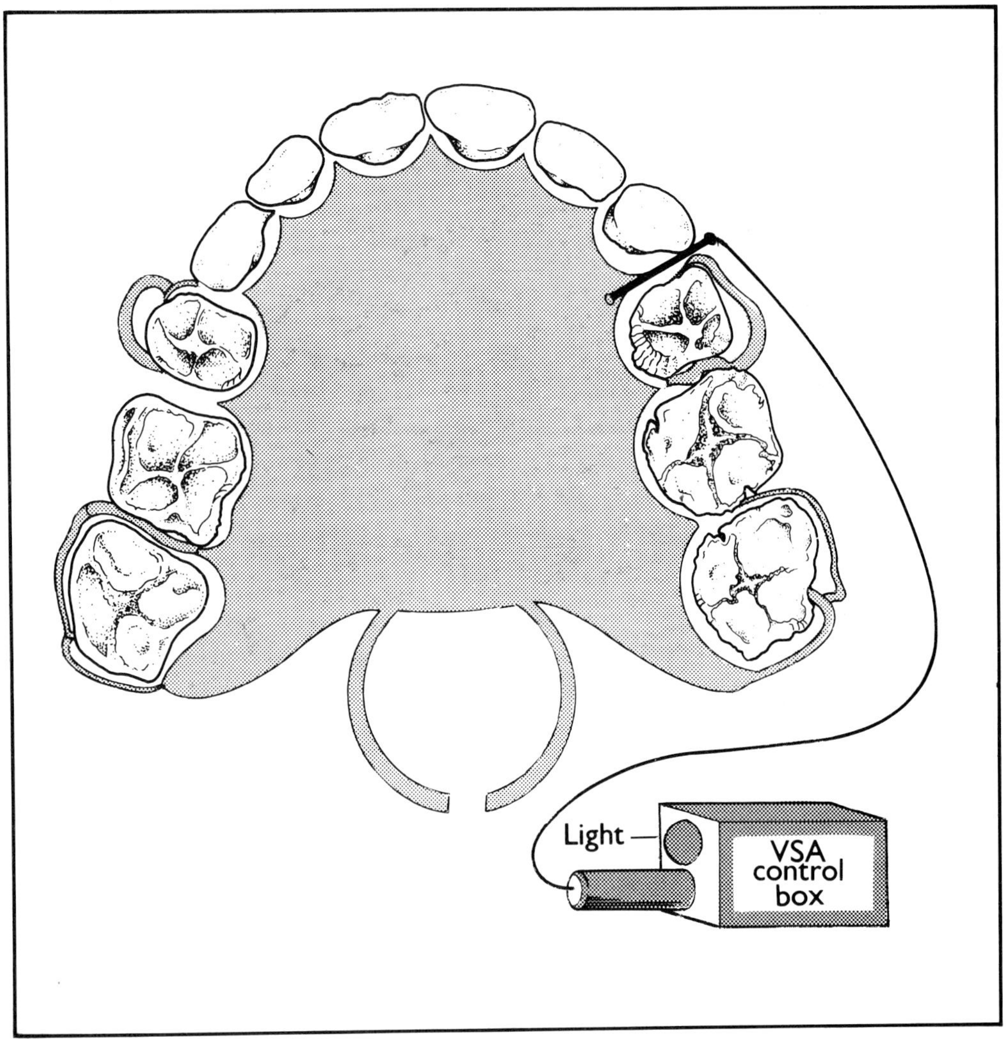

Figure 9.3 ***Visual speech aid***

Design Modification

Some patients find difficulties in the use of the VSA because the circuit sometimes remains completed by mucus across the electrodes, even though the soft palate is raised. Some centres have therefore modified the design of the electrodes. At the Birmingham Dental Hospital in the UK the author has found the most reliable modification to be the one shown in *Figure 9.4*. Here one electrode is placed above the other. The upper one, which contacts the soft palate, is made of very springy stainless wire which, when the soft palate is raised, quickly bounces off the lower electrode to ensure that the circuit is broken.

Where these aids are fitted in a specialist unit, but regular treatment is carried out in the client's home locality, the clinician responsible for the treatment would find it beneficial to visit the unit to discuss the design and use of the appliances.

Evaluation of Progress

With the use of both the PTA and the VSA careful records should be kept through audio-recording to monitor progress. An initial period of treatment should be agreed, with sufficient time to achieve change; three months is suggested. If at review there is no evidence of progress, the anatomical proportions of the velopharyngeal mechanism should again be questioned and further investigated.

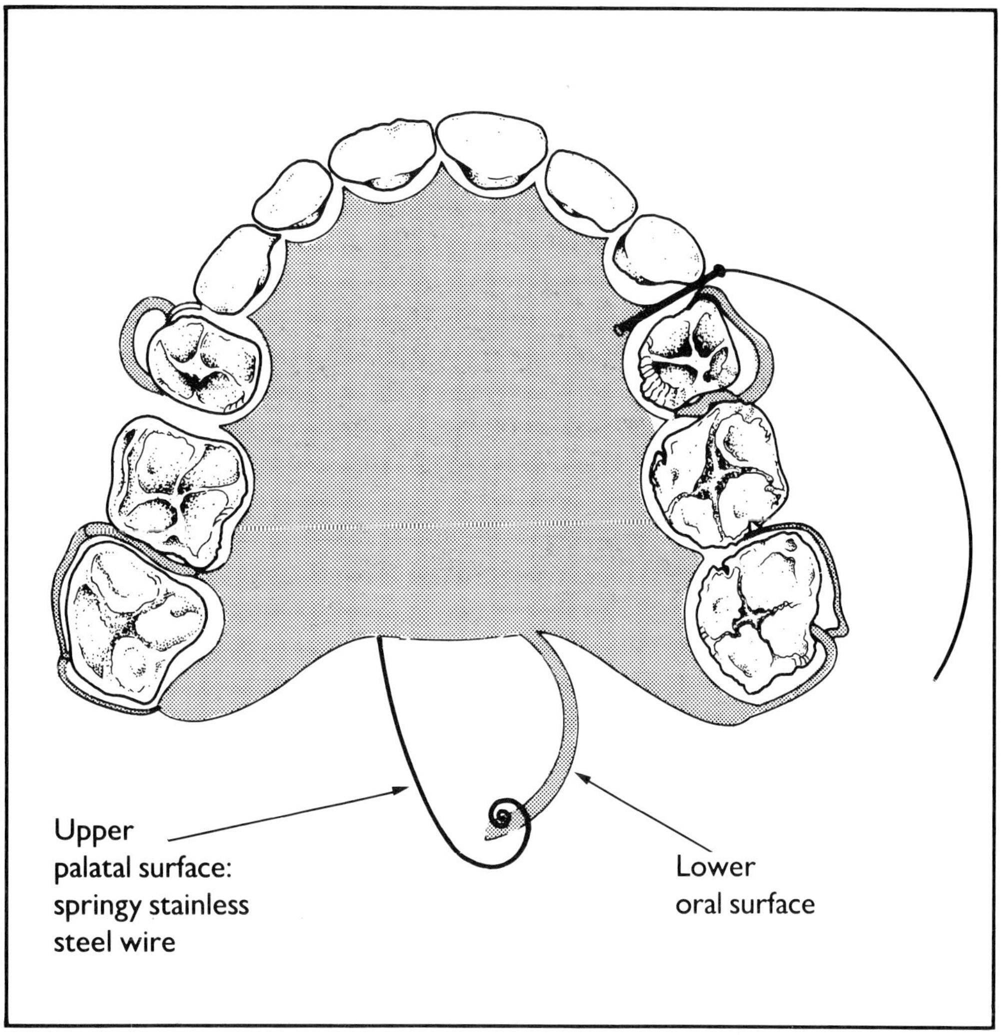

Figure 9.4 ***Modified design for electrodes for VSA***

Cost-effectiveness

Both the PTA and VSA are comparatively inexpensive pieces of equipment which, if correctly prescribed, may bring about speech change which cannot be effected by any other means. Progress can be accelerated and the period of intervention reduced. The PTA promotes improved function of the soft palate throughout the time it is worn, while the VSA allows frequent and independent practice without the speech clinician being present. The role of the clinician is to give instruction in use, to enable the patient to understand the relationship between the feedback, the function of the soft palate and speech and to give suitable graded exercises to be undertaken regularly. The use of these appliances is therefore evident in cost-effective terms. The control box for the VSA is reusable, so that a general department with a mixed case load could manage with two control boxes.

Electropalatography (EPG)

EPG is described here because, although it is expensive in terms of computer hardware, the appliance worn by the patient is relatively inexpensive and is likely to become cheaper. The computer hardware may already be available in the department, or accessible elsewhere. With some patients the use of EPG may provide a breakthrough to progress and therefore must be considered as one of the possible treatment procedures. It can be of particular value in those cases where deviant speech patterns are deeply entrenched and not amenable to conventional remedial procedures. These may be cases where speech intervention has already been provided over long periods of time with little or no improvement. EPG differs from the PTA and VSA in that the focus is on tongue to hard palate contacts, which are frequently markedly deviant in articulatory patterns of cleft palate cases. The introduction of EPG can provide the essential feedback on tongue to hard palate contacts to effect change in deviant patterns, as well as providing an important motivation to patients and clinician where further improvement seems almost impossible. With older children, teenagers and adults the use of EPG may be very acceptable because of the technology used, taking the pressure off the clinician–client interaction as part of the treatment process.

EPG has been used with a wide range of patients. The system described here is the one developed in the UK at the University of Reading (**Hardcastle**, 1984). **Hardcastle *et al*** (1989) have described the use of EPG with two cleft palate cases. It can be used as both an assessment and a treatment tool. Slightly different systems are developing in some other countries.

The Equipment

The 'palate'

The acrylic plate worn by the patient for EPG, usually termed the 'palate', is individually made. It extends from the alveolar ridge to the margin of the hard palate. Embedded in the acrylic palate are 62 electrodes (*see Figure 9.5*) arranged in a predetermined pattern, according to anatomical landmarks. The placing of the electrodes may be difficult where the maxilla is very narrow and highly arched. The electrodes are exposed on the lingual surface so that, when contacted by the tongue, a circuit is completed. Wires lead out of the mouth from the palate to the processing unit and from there to the microcomputer. The palate is worn only for practice purposes.

If the patient has not worn a plate previously a trainer plate must be provided, to be worn for gradually longer periods until it can be tolerated for 24 hours and speech becomes adjusted to wear (**Hardcastle *et al***, 1989). For construction of the palate good impressions need to be taken by the dental specialist. Some centres are able to construct their own palates, but usually these are sent away for expert preparation.

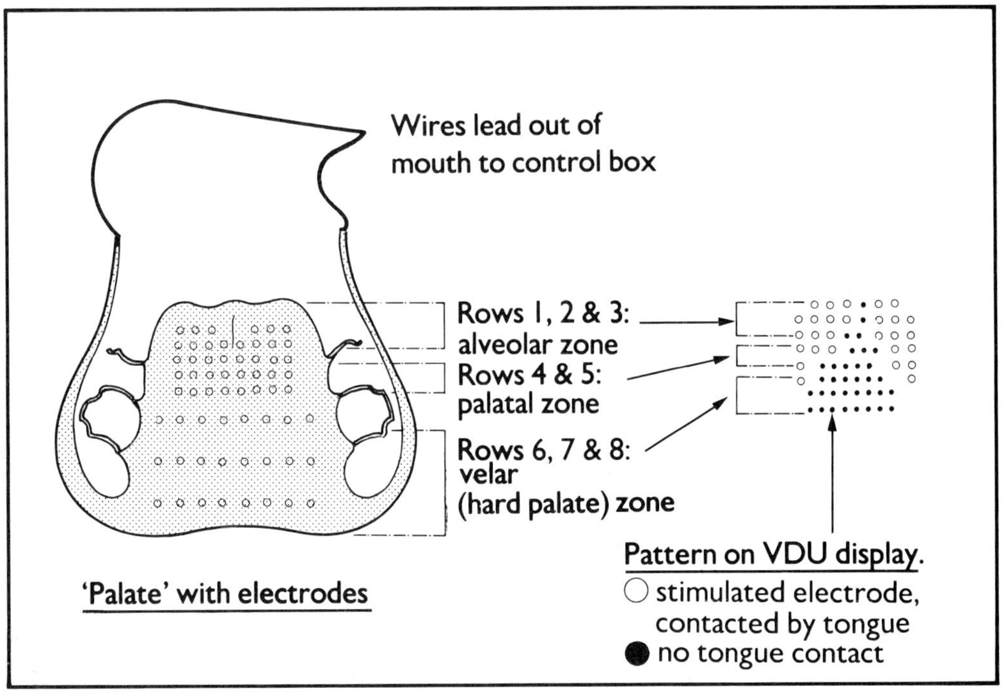

Figure 9.5 ***Electropalatography***

The processing unit

Signals from the electrodes are passed out of the mouth via a processing unit and shown on the visual display unit (VDU) of the microcomputer. The contacts are displayed in a schematic form representing the layout of the electrodes in the palate. As the tongue contacts an electrode this lights up on the screen, showing contacts every 10 milliseconds. The pattern can be frozen at any point, for analysis. For each phoneme a number of contacts are made. Research with normal speakers provides typical patterns of contact for a range of phonemes. The temporal pattern of contacts shows how the pattern of contacts changes as the sound is produced. Although in normal speakers each individual shows slightly different patterns of contact, there is enough similarity to provide a target pattern. If the clinician wears a palate this can be displayed with a split-screen facility to provide a model for the client.

The information fed into the computer can be produced in the form of a print-out. The procedure can therefore be used in continuing therapy or for later analysis from the print-out. The analysis of the print-out is extremely time-consuming and therefore not usually possible for clinicians other than for research purposes. However some analysis is essential to examine the contacts in different phonetic contexts. This is important as improved contacts in some contexts may provide the way to achieving change.

Use in Treatment

If EPG is introduced to help a patient have insight into tongue–palate contacts they will need to have access to the equipment on a frequent basis if change is to be effected.

Suitable Cases

1 Cases should be selected where the main speech difficulties are at the articulatory/phonetic level. Improvement in resonance is not likely to result from the use of EPG, other than the general overall improvement in speech acceptability which results from phonetic improvement. Decrease in perceived nasality is associated with greater use of final consonants.

2 Individuals must be:

(a) old enough to tolerate having impressions and able to co-operate with the fitting and wearing of the palate — wearing the training plate will establish this;

(b) mature enough to use the system;

(c) intellectually capable of understanding the feedback;

(d) motivated to use the system;

(e) able to attend on a frequent and regular basis.

If EPG can be introduced at the optimum time, months of ineffective treatment may be saved, so that expensive equipment can reduce the clinician time.

Availability

EPG is not likely to be easily available to most clinicians, primarily because of the need for a suitable microcomputer. Its use with cleft palate cases is now well established. This, together with the fact that it can also be used with a wide range of other cases, for example for dysarthrias, dyspraxia and phonological problems, makes it a more feasible technology for general departments. The support of a dental department is essential. The microcomputer may also be used with other procedures.

Nasendoscopy

Nasendoscopy, designed as an assessment tool, provides feedback on the status of the velopharyngeal sphincter through video display and could therefore be used in treatment. Micronose is an example of the available biofeedback instrumentation. In cases where velopharyngeal closure is stimulable, this therapeutic approach is being explored with success (**Witzel *et al***, 1989). Liaison with the specialist speech therapist regarding the availability of this treatment is recommended.

Suppliers of Equipment

Electropalatography

Linguistics Department, The University of Reading, Whiteknights, Reading, Berks RG6 2AA, England. Distributed by Migrant Wells Limited, PO Box 3, 7 Stanley Road, Rugby CV21 3UF.

Nasal Anemometer, PTA and VSA

Bio Instrumentation Limited, Holm Croft, Silverton, Exeter EX5 4JH, England.

Micronose

SCI Instruments, 39 Hinton Way, Great Shelford, Cambridge CB2 5AX, England.

CHAPTER 10
CASE EXAMPLES

A Period of Therapy in a Young Child/*102*
Speech and Language Assessment at Three Years/*102*
Examination of the Speech Mechanism/*103*
The Problems/*103*
Intervention Plan/*104*
Methods of Intervention/*104*
Treatment of a Teenager with an Unrepaired Palate Cleft/*105*
Speech Assessment/*106*
Information from School/*106*
Achieving Improved Communication/*106*
Progress/*107*
Working with an Adult/*108*
Speech Assessment/*109*
Progress/*110*

CHAPTER 10
CASE EXAMPLES

A Period of Therapy in a Young Child

Jeremy, aged three years, is presented to illustrate the nature of the speech problems in a young child, the overall management, planning intervention and methods adopted. Jeremy's case is summarised in *Figure 10.1*. The case is not atypical, presenting many problems which the clinician may need to tackle.

> Jeremy was born with a complete unilateral cleft of lip and palate.
>
> He had his lip repaired at four months and his palate repaired in two stages: the soft palate at four months and the hard palate at two years and ten months. A very small oro-nasal fistula remained just behind the alveolus.
>
> There was a history of hearing loss with myringotomies carried out at two years and nine months.

Figure 10.1 ***Case outline: Jeremy, three years***

Speech and Language Assessment at Three Years

Language evaluation using the Reynell Developmental Language Scales and the analysis of data using Language Assessment, Remediation and Screening Procedure (LARSP) (**Crystal *et al*,** 1976) indicated that language was developing adequately, although there had been some concern earlier. In the clinical context Jeremy tended to use one-word utterances. He was reported to be socially well-integrated and now willing to talk in most situations. Connected speech was sometimes unintelligible.

Speech evaluation revealed:

- Marked hypernasality;
- Nasal emission;
- Reduced volume;
- Deviant articulation;
- A reduced phonological system.

The phonetic inventory was limited, consisting of:

/m/m̥/n/n̥/ŋ/ɱ/h/l/j/ϑ/ʔ/.

The observations of speech can be summarised as follows:

1 The phonetic inventory was severely reduced.
2 All vowels nasalised but correct otherwise.
3 All final consonants, except nasals, deleted or glottalised.
4 Many oral sounds realised as homorganic nasals, although place sometimes changed; eg. fish ⟶ [nĩ].
5 Many medial and final consonants replaced by [ʔ].
6 Occasional voicing confusions occurred; eg. key ⟶ [ñi].
7 Not all realisations stable.
8 Some evidence of ability to produce velars; eg. singing ⟶[n̥ɪnɪŋ].
9 Approximants, which require minimal constriction of the vocal tract, present but not always used contrastively.
10 The only plosive /ʔ/.
11 Voiceless nasals used in an attempt to signal phonological contrasts; eg. for /s/ and /t/ > [n̥] and /p/ > [m̥].

Examination of the Speech Mechanism

Examination of the peripheral speech mechanism showed the following:

1 Normal dentition and occlusion for age.
2 Small oro-nasal fistula.
3 Soft palate appeared somewhat short and not very mobile on /a:/.
4 Occasional nasal regurgitation was reported with some thin substances.

The Problems

Jeremy's case throws up a number of problems for the team and the speech clinician. The following points should be considered:

1 The hard palate was repaired only two months before the assessment.
2 Patterns of pre-operative speech persist.
3 What might be the significance of the fistula, as opposed to the velopharyngeal mechanism?
4 What would normally be expected in the speech of an English-speaking child at aged three years? The phonetic inventory would usually include: /m,n,h,w,y,p,b,k,g,t,d,f/ and possibly /r,l/. Comparing this with Jeremy's inventory, there is an outstanding lack of plosion within the mouth; /l/ is present while /w/ is not.
5 The phonological processes expected at this stage would be cluster reduction and final consonant deletion. Examples of consonant deletion can be found in:

   gate ⟶[nẽĩ],
   mug ⟶[mʌ̃].

   Fronting which should be reducing is evident in:

   key ⟶[ñi:],
   gate ⟶[nẽĩ].

   However, although the speech samples can be looked at from a phonological perspective, it is evident that the springboard is one of difficulty in sound production. Describing the problem within a phonological framework may not be of help in the remedial process. There are indications that Jeremy is aware of and attempting to make phonological contrasts (*see page 103, no. 11*).

6 What is the dominant tongue position? Could it possibly be held high in the mouth to stop air passing into the fistula? Note, in this context, the late repair of the hard palate, which may have had an effect on tongue posture.

7 The only fricative present is the glottal /h/. Does this relate to inadequacy of the velopharyngeal sphincter or is /h/ used because pre-operatively air was bound to pass into the nose through the open hard palate and friction could therefore only be produced at the glottis?

8 What is the status of the structures as a basis for articulatory placement?

9 What is the role of the hearing impairment in relation to speech?

Intervention Plan

Jeremy is three years old, with severe speech difficulties. Language development indicates that he is of at least average intellectual potential. He is too young for nasendoscopy to establish the potential adequacy of the velopharyngeal mechanism. Although he only had his hard palate repaired at two years ten months, it would be unwise to allow time to elapse as he may retain pre-operative patterns, which will be maintained through auditory feedback. It would be helpful to know what expectations the parents had of the operation in relation to speech. It is to be hoped that an immediate speech change was not anticipated.

It is important to try to establish (a) if speech can be improved with help and (b) the status of the velopharyngeal sphincter. A period of diagnostic therapy should be implemented. The willingness of the parents to attend for a regular period, once weekly over six months, and to work with Jeremy each day needs to be established. The aims of intervention, as suggested in *Figure 10.2*, should be agreed with the parents. Members of the team should be made aware of the management plan.

1	To increase awareness, sensitivity and mobility of oral structures as a basis for extension of phonetic inventory.
2	To ensure that the recognition and discrimination of sounds is adequate as a basis for production.
3	To explore sound stimulability in order to identify which sounds may be most easily achieved.
4	To explore the possible significance of the oro-nasal fistula, although size would indicate that it is not significant.
5	To improve sound production in one consonant as a way into further work.
6	To achieve the production of some consonants (at least up to CV level) which require a high level of intra-oral pressure, ie plosives/fricatives.

Figure 10.2 ***Aims of a diagnostic period of therapy for Jeremy***

Methods of Intervention

The value of setting out the aims and matching the methods to them cannot be over-emphasised. The mother should be present throughout the sessions, to learn new procedures and to demonstrate what progress has been made at home.

Methodology

1 Increase awareness and sensitivity of structures — follow programme as described on *pages 69–70*.

2 Follow procedures for auditory discrimination and recognition.

3 Keep hearing under review, through reports and clinical observation. Refer to ENT if necessary.

4 Assess stimulability of the whole range of consonants which should be possible at age three years. Imitation should be used as well as procedures to increase feedback and awareness such as demonstration of air-stream, feeling, mirror. Stimulability should be recorded and reviewed at monthly intervals.

5 Stimulability should also be undertaken while the fistula is obturated with dental wax. This should only be done in clinic and should be carefully supervised. If the main source of nasal emission is the fistula, obturation should reduce it. If it does not reduce then the velopharyngeal sphincter is more likely to be responsible, although strong habits cannot be ruled out.

6 Work on a sound which Jeremy is not likely to find too difficult. It should be selected on the following basis:

- Stimulability;
- Developmental expectations;
- Easy to teach because visible and easily demonstrated;
- Not requiring high-level intra-oral air pressure.

Taking these factors into account /w/ might be selected: it is visible and would easily lead on from the exercises to increase flexibility of lip movement.

7 The stimulability test should indicate which pressure consonant should be selected. This can be introduced while work on /w/ continues. In line with normal development, plosives should be attempted first. However, if they trigger the glottal plosive, they may have to be left. The fricative /f/ might be preferred because developmentally it should be present; it is easily visible and unlikely to trigger the glottal.

The sound selected will need to be established in isolation, in CV, VC and CVC combinations, using a range of vowels. (High vowels are more nasalised and may need to be avoided.) Work should be done on nonsense words free of laid-down patterns locked into the semantic, before moving on to known words. Progress with a pressure consonant is essential in the diagnostic process. Procedures for eliciting new sounds are suggested in *Figures 8.7*, *8.8* and *8.9*.

Treatment of a Teenager with an Unrepaired Palate Cleft

Karen was born with a cleft lip and a large 'U'-shaped cleft of hard and soft palate. The lip was repaired in infancy but Karen was left with a very small pre-maxilla and tight, scarred upper lip. Her palate was not repaired because there was not enough tissue to effect a repair. Karen also had a deformity of the right hand.

Karen was referred to speech therapy at 14 years of age by the orthodontist. Speech help had not been provided before, nor had it been sought previously, but Karen indicated that she was conscious about her speech and wanted help. There was a history of poor family support for the management offered and this was why speech help had not been provided earlier.

Speech Assessment

Assessment at referral showed the following features:

- Marked hypernasality;
- Nasal emission;
- Tendency to nasal grimace;
- Poor breath support;
- Low volume;
- Excessive speed of utterance;
- Weakened fricatives and plosives;
- Velars absent;
- All clusters poor, with /s/ clusters presenting marked difficulty;
- Variable intelligibility; specific to some words which presented articulation problems, and general, especially in new social situations.

Information from School

Contact with school showed that Karen was of average potential but was under-achieving. She attended a special unit for physically handicapped children, but was reluctant to attend the mainstream unit, although opportunities were being provided for her to do so. There had been some difficulties about school attendance, but no other behavioural difficulties. She was noted to be self-conscious about her appearance and was often reluctant to communicate. Karen was particularly self-conscious about eating and did not like anyone to watch her. This was probably a major factor in her reluctance to go into mainstream school.

Discussion with Karen showed that she was very aware of her poor communication and was motivated to improve. However she had very little insight into the nature of and reasons for her difficulties.

Achieving Improved Communication

General management

1. Referral was made back to the plastic surgeon regarding the possibility of repair to her palate, but this was still not possible.
2. Karen was already wearing an obturator, which only covered the hard palate cleft. Discussion with the orthodontist led to a decision that the obturator should be extended as far back as possible into the velopharynx, with the hope of impeding some of the direct air-flow up into the nasal passages, and of providing an articulation contact for velars.
3. A period of treatment was provided.

Treatment aims

Treatment aims (*see Figure 10.3*) concentrated on those aspects where improvement was considered to be possible; for example, although consonant clusters were a problem of which Karen was aware and concerned, they were not considered an appropriate area to work on in the context of the physical limitations. Karen attended on a weekly basis, which was considered sufficient because she needed to understand that change would be brought about primarily by her own efforts. Furthermore she would not miss too much schooling. Family support was limited, but a visit to school helped in enlisting co-operation and encouragement. It was evident that, although sympathetic, the school had virtually no understanding of the nature and cause of her speech difficulties.

1	Help Karen to achieve a greater awareness of the components of speaking and how these might be improved in her own speech.
2	Improve the breath support for speech.
3	Encourage 'open' relaxed communication with particular attention to paralinguistic features such as eye contact and attention to the listener.
4	Achieve speech production with increased mouth opening to encourage maximum oral air-stream.
5	Increase volume.
6	Reduce speed.
7	If appropriate and possible, introduce specific work on articulation; for example, velars might be possible with the extension to the obturator.

Figure 10.3 **Aims of treatment for Karen**

Individual sessions

Figure 10.4 shows a plan for an individual session early on in Karen's treatment, while *Figure 10.5* shows a session a month later. Procedures such as self-rating scales were introduced early on in therapy to ensure that Karen could monitor her own attempts when working independently.

Progress

Karen worked hard and generally attended her appointments. Improvement was made over a period of a year's treatment, when it ceased because of other demands on her, including the possibility of a further education course. Karen had become generally more confident about her communication. This, together with some reduction in speed and willingness to speak more loudly and the use of wider mouth opening, made her speech more intelligible and acceptable to the listener because of a slight reduction in nasality and nasal emission, achieved by a more relaxed approach to speaking. A velar-type sound was achieved. This was imprecise and slightly affricated and she did not always manage to use it in connected speech, but she could use it if it was important to intelligibility.

Although the palate remained unrepaired, a good fitting was obtained for the obturator which was also used to carry incisors. The fitting of dentures made a marked improvement in Karen's appearance and increased her confidence.

	AIMS	METHODS
1	Establish if homework was done and if this was found helpful.	Talk about practice done at home; identify problems.
2	Establish if relaxation was done and if it was helpful.	Discussion and demonstration.
3	Explore posture and breath support. Establish Karen's level of awareness of her own posture and breathing in preparation for self-monitoring.	Discussion and demonstration. Encourage to reflect on self.
4	Improvement of posture and mouth opening.	Use of mirror to see if it helps and is acceptable. Practise short sentences with increased mouth opening.
5	Improvement in level and monitoring of relaxation.	Use tape to see if it can be used at home. Relax and encourage Karen to monitor. Discuss relationship to speech.
6	Establish greater insight into Karen's own speech, especially the importance of volume and speed in achieving intelligibility.	Tape conversation, listen to and discuss. Direct Karen's attention to aspects which can be attended to in treatment.
7	Plan work to be carried out in week and ensure that Karen has full understanding of what she has to do.	From insight achieved in 6, select areas for attention. Give clear instructions for work to be done on audio-tape with demonstrations where appropriate, eg. speed.

Figure 10.4 **Session plan for Karen: I**

Karen's management illustrates the value of providing treatment, even in situations where the eventual speech outcome is likely to be limited. The results could make all the difference to her future. The treatment plan adopted illustrates the importance of tackling a wide range of aspects of disordered communication and not focusing too much on the articulation, which, if tackled 'head on', might only lead to failure.

Working with an Adult

Mr N (45 years) was referred by the prosthetic specialist. Mr N was having dentures fitted and had asked if help for his speech was available. He reported that he was ridiculed about his speech, had recently lost his job and felt that his poor speech would put him at a disadvantage in getting further employment. He was considerably depressed. In his job as a security officer in a factory he used his speech for telephoning and using a walkie-talkie.

	AIMS	METHODS
1	Evaluate the usefulness of school visit in Karen's view (visit taken place previous day); Karen present throughout the discussion.	Discussion re visit, future needs, therapy plan etc. Karen's feelings.
2	Evaluation of home practice on volume and speed.	Listen to tape made of role play done with sister. Split tape into sections for evaluation. Use five-point scale for evaluation of volume and speed.
3	Carryover of improvements into everyday situations.	Role play with friend Karen has brought to clinic. Role play of ordering meal at McDonalds. Video and evaluate using rating scale.
4	Increase awareness of communication in general.	Re-look at video, paying attention to posture and eye contact.
5	Set assignments for week.	Select role play from Karen's suggestions, to be done with friend and evaluated.

Figure 10.5 **Session plan for Karen: II (one month after session plan I)**

His palate had been repaired in infancy and again when he was 30; the nature of the second operation was not clear. He had received some speech therapy following this operation. Examination of the speech mechanism showed that the soft palate was extremely short. (He had asked the prosthetic specialist if he could have a uvula.) A large oro-nasal fistula remained in the hard palate. An acrylic plate was to be fitted which would obturate the fistula and carry dentures, which he had not worn before.

Speech Assessment

Initial speech assessment showed the following:

- Occasional unintelligibility;
- Marked hypernasality;
- Some audible nasal emission, especially accompanying and masking the attempted /s/;
- /k/g/ very difficult because of lack of velum;
- Could produce most consonants in isolation, except /k/g/;
- Alveolars poorly articulated in connected speech;
- Plosives weakened and accompanied by glottal;
- Fricatives weak;
- Constant use of hard glottal attack;
- Excessive speed of utterance; as rate increased, intelligibility decreased;
- /s/ clusters were poorly articulated;
- Mr N's speech tended to be very dysfluent, almost amounting to

stammer: he spoke with considerable tension; with increased tension, speech became rapid, forced and unintelligible;

- His understanding of speech and insight into his own difficulties were extremely limited.

Informal observations, followed by audiometric screening, indicated that hearing loss was present. A letter was sent to the ENT consultant, requesting further information. The presence of a perforated right ear-drum was reported, as well as some hearing loss in the left ear.

Treatment aims

Discussion with Mr N showed that he was highly motivated to achieve some improvement in his speech. It was decided to offer a trial period of treatment following the fitting of his new dentures. The aims of the treatment are shown in *Figure 10.6*.

1	To increase awareness of speech production and of the difficulties in patient's own speech.
2	To improve intelligibility by: decreasing rate; Boone open mouth technique. Introduce self-monitoring as soon as possible.
3	Decrease hard glottal attack, by making Mr N aware of what hard glottal attack is. May be helped by open mouth technique and reduced tension; if not, use Boone elimination of hard glottal attack programme.
4	Improve general articulation by increasing awareness of tongue placement; increase sensory awareness by PNF techniques. Use articulatory diagrams. Use plate for awareness of contacts at alveolar ridge.
5	Promote a more relaxed approach to speaking with increased intelligibility and confidence.
(See **Boone DR,** *Voice Program for Adults*, 1982.)	

Figure 10.6 ***Aims of intervention, Mr N***

Progress

Over a nine-month period Mr N made considerable progress with his speech, while there was a marked gain in confidence. Rate slowed and fluency increased. The reduced tension in speaking had modified but not eliminated the hard glottal attack. There was improvement in the precision of articulation of alveolars. The plate was considered to be of importance here, as it heightened the awareness of the intra-oral environment. His /s/ clusters showed some improvement, but still needed a lot of care — he could use them in slow, careful speech. During the treatment period Mr N got another job. (An example of a treatment session is shown in *Figure 10.7*.)

The period of treatment was considered to be extremely worthwhile, and although speech problems (particularly hypernasality) persisted, the improvement in certain aspects helped Mr N accept some limitations inevitable in the context of his physical difficulties, especially as he was aware of his increased intelligibility, which reduced anxiety about speaking.

This case serves to illustrate the value of treatment even into middle life. The provision of the dentures was considered to be a key to articulatory improvement, as it changed the intra-oral environment and therefore enhanced Mr N's awareness of tongue-tip to alveolar ridge and palate contacts. In addition he worked assiduously on his speech, always carrying out work given in the sessions, and showing marked progress in his awareness and self-monitoring.

	AIMS	METHODS
1	Investigate use of open mouth.	Review open mouth technique, go over home practice, check rating charts. Repetition of sentences for open mouth technique. Mr N to describe picture, using open mouth technique. Spontaneous speech using above.
2	Increase awareness of voiced/ voiceless contrasts.	Explain voiced/voiceless contrast using diagrams, feeling larynx etc. Get Mr N to explain the concept to the student who is present. Discrimination tasks with pairs of sounds and initially in words.
3	To improve self-monitoring and production of /s/ clusters.	Go through 'build-up' cards used at home: /oon//poon// spoon/. When the problem is approached in this way, Mr N finds it easier to include all the elements, and by practising the vowel first reduces the tendency to use a glottal for /p/. Encourage self-evaluation of production.
4	Carryover of improvements to connected speech and increase in intelligibility.	Describing people in magazine, listener to enquire when anything is unintelligible. Listener to identify topic of description.

Figure 10.7 ***Session plan for Mr N***

APPENDIX I
ORO-FACIAL EXAMINATION

Name __________	**DOB** __________	**Sex** __________
Age at assessment ______	**Date** __________	**Number** __________
Materials	Surgical gloves Mouth examination mirror Spatula Pen torch	Tissues Glass of water Cotton buds Crisps/biscuits

Tick heading as appropriate

NOSE				
1	Shape	normal	flattened	deflected
2	Breathing	nasal	oral	mixed
3	Ability to blow nose	yes	no	
4	Nasal grimace	none	mild	severe
MOUTH OPENING				
1	Size of opening	normal	microstomia	macrostomia
2	Degree of opening	normal	restricted	
LIPS				
1	Competence	normal	incompetent	variable
2	Balance	normal	poor	
3	Upper lip	normal	scarred	tight
4	Lower lip	normal	full	tight
5	Function in speech	normal	adequate	restricted
6	Function in swallowing	normal	open	excessive
7	Function in feeding	normal	flaccid	excessive
8	Drooling	none	mild/moderate	severe
TONGUE				
1	Size in relation to dental arches	normal	large	small
2	Crenation	none	yes	
3	Symmetry on protrusion	normal	asymmetrical	
4	Appearance of tongue-tip on protrusion	normal	excessive/ uncontrolled	limited
5	Length of frenum	normal	short	
6	Activity in speech	normal	fronted	limited

7	Elevation to alveolar ridge	normal	adequate	poor
8	General movement	normal	weak	unco-ordinated
HARD PALATE				
1	Pre-maxilla	normal	cleft	
2	Alveolar ridge	normal	scarred	cleft
3	Scarring	none	mild	severe
4	Sensitivity	good	adequate	poor
5	Fistula	none	small	large
6	Colour	normal	blue zone	
7	Contour	normal	narrow	wide
8	Depth	normal	high	shallow
SOFT PALATE				
1	Intact	yes	no	
2	Uvula	intact	bifid	other
3	Length	normal	short	
4	Mobility	normal	moderate	poor
5	Scarring	none	mild	severe
6	Activity in speech	normal	hyponasal	hypernasal
7	Movement on phonation	normal	poor	absent
8	Sensitivity	normal	hyposensitive	hypersensitive
NASOPHARYNX				
1	Depth	normal	deep	restricted
2	Movement of pillars	normal	poor	absent
3	Tonsils: size	visible	small	large
4	Tonsils: infected	no	mild	severe
DENTITION/OCCLUSION				
1	Pre-maxilla	normal	small	prognathic
2	Maxilla	normal	small	prognathic
3	Incisors	normal	forward absent	overjet
4	Skeletal relationship of maxilla/mandible	normal	class II	class III
5	Open bite	none	mild	severe
6	Dentition	normal	crowding	missing
7	Oral hygiene	good	adequate	poor
8	Appliance	none	removable	fixed

APPENDIX II
DIAGNOSTIC RATING CHECKLIST

Name ______________________________ **DOB** __________
Date of referral ______________________________ **Date** __________

Rate 0 for a poor feature and 6 for a positive feature. It is recognised that not all features have the same significance for prognosis; however it is extremely difficult to identify which features will be of major consequence in any individual case.

	FEATURES	**RATING/SCORE**
		0 1 2 3 4 5 6
1	Delay in diagnosing condition (no delay = 6, long delay = 0)	
2	Severity of original condition (severe = 0/1, mild = 5/6)	
3	Timing of surgery (not undertaken = 0, optimum = 6)	
4	Adequacy of velopharyngeal mechanism	
5	Status of larynx	
6	Dental and occlusal status	
7	Status of speech	
8	Degree of speech change with treatment	
9	Length of time in which speech standard has not improved (long time = 0)	
10	Status of language	
11	Hearing status	
12	Possibility of remediating hearing loss (if hearing loss not present = 6)	
13	Intellectual potential	
14	Adjustment of individual to communication	
15	Awareness of individual to communication difficulties in general	
16	Awareness and insight of individual into specific speech difficulties	
17	Presence/absence of other physical limitations	
18	Availability of speech therapy	
19	Appropriateness of speech therapy provision, ie clinician experience and availability	
20	Family support and adjustment	
21	Availability of other support to carry out day-to-day work if necessary. Or self-motivation of adult.	
	FULL SCORE = 126	**TOTAL**

APPENDIX III
USEFUL ADDRESSES

AFASIC — The Association for all Speech-impaired Children
347 Central Markets, Smithfield, London EC1A 9NH

American Cleft Palate Educational Foundation
University of Pittsburgh, 331 Salk Hall, Pittsburgh, Pennsylvania 15261

CLAPA — Cleft Lip and Palate Association
1, Eastwood Gardens, Kenton, Newcastle upon Tyne, NE3 3DQ

College of Speech Therapists
Harold Poster House, 6 Lechmere Road, London NW2 5BU

The Cranio-facial Society
c/o AG Huddart, Consultant Orthodontist, The Corbett Hospital, Vicarage Road, Amblecote, Stourbridge, West Midlands DY8 4JB

VOCAL — Voluntary Organisations Communication and Language
336 Brixton Road, London SW9 7AA

BIBLIOGRAPHY

Albery L, 'Approaches to the Treatment of Speech Problems', Stengelhofen J (ed), *Cleft Palate: The Nature and Remediation of Communication Problems*, Churchill Livingstone, Edinburgh, 1989.

Albery L & Enderby P, 'Intensive Speech Therapy with Cleft Palate Children', *British Journal of Disorders of Communication*, 19, p2, 1984.

Anthony A, Bogle D, Ingram TTS & McIsaac MW, *Edinburgh Articulation Test*, Churchill Livingstone, Edinburgh, 1971.

Barrett RH & Hanson ML, *Oral Myofunctional Disorders*, CV Mosby & Co, St Louis, 1978.

Boone DR, *The Voice and Voice Therapy*, 2nd edn, Prentice Hall, New Jersey, 1977.

Boone DR, *Voice Program for Adults*, CC Publications, Oregon, 1982.

Brookshire BL, Lynch JI & Fox DR, *A Parent–child Cleft Palate Curriculum: Developing Speech and Language*, CC Publications, Oregon, 1980.

Bzoch KR (ed), *Communication Disorders Related to Cleft Lip and Palate*, 2nd edn, Little Brown & Co, Boston, Mass, 1979.

Canning BAM & Rose MF, 'Clinical Measurement of the Speed of Tongue and Lip Movements in British Children with Normal Speech', *British Journal of Disorders of Communication*, 9, p1, 1974.

The Cleft Palate Unit, *Your Cleft Lip and Palate Child. A Guide for Parents*, Frenchay Hospital, Bristol, date not known.

Cooke J & Williams D, *Working with Children's Language*, Winslow Press, Bicester, 1985.

Cooper H, Harding R, Crogman W, Mazaheri M & Millard R, *Cleft Lip and Cleft Palate: A Team Approach to Management*, WB Saunders & Co, Philadelphia, 1979.

Crystal D, *An Introduction to Language Pathology*, Edward Arnold, London, 1980.

Crystal D, Fletcher P & Garman M, *The Grammatical Analysis of Language Disability*, Edward Arnold, London, 1976.

Curle HJ, 'Therapeutic Methods for the Incompetent Soft Palate', Ellis RE & Flack FC (eds), *Diagnosis and Treatment of Palatoglossal Malfunction*, The College of Speech Therapists, London, 1979.

Edwards M & Watson ACH (eds), *Advances in the Management of Cleft Palate*, Churchill Livingstone, Edinburgh, 1980.

Elbert M & Gierut J, *Handbook of Clinical Phonology*, Taylor & Francis, London, 1986.

Ellis RE, Flack FC, Curle HJ & Selley WG, 'A System for the Assessment of Nasal Airflow During Speech', *British Journal of Disorders of Communication*, 13, p1, 1978.

Enderby P. & Philipp R, 'Speech and Language Handicap: Towards Knowing the Size of the Problem', *British Journal of Disorders of Communication*, 21, p2, 1986.

Fawcus M (ed), *Voice Disorders and their Management*, Croom Helm, Beckenham, 1986.

Fletcher SG, *Diagnosing Speech Problems from Cleft Palate*, Grune & Stratton, New York, 1972.

Fletcher SG, *Time-by-count Test of Diadochokinetic Syllable Rate*, CC Publications, Oregon, 1978.

Foster TD, 'The Role of Orthodontic Treatment', Edwards M & Watson ACH (eds), *Advances in the Management of Cleft Palate*, Churchill Livingstone, Edinburgh, 1980.

Frey BJ, *Tongue Position Charts*, Winslow Press, Bicester, 1987.

Goldman R, Fristoe M & Woodcock MM, *Test of Auditory Discrimination*, American Guidance Service, Minnesota, 1970.

Goldman R & Fristoe M, *Goldman–Fristoe Test of Articulation*, AGS Inc, Minnesota, 1972.

Gorlin RJ, Pindborg JJ & Cohen MM, *Syndromes of the Head and Neck*, McGraw Hill, New York, 1976.

Grunwell P, *Clinical Phonology*, Croom Helm, London & Sydney, 1982.

Grunwell P (ed), *The Phonetic Representation of Disordered Speech*, Project Paper No. 38, King's Fund, London, 1983.

Grunwell P, *Phonological Assessment of Child Speech (PACS)*, NFER/ Nelson, Windsor, 1985.

Grunwell P & Russell J, 'Vocalisations Before and After Cleft Palate Surgery: A Pilot Study', *British Journal of Disorders of Communication*, 22, p1, 1987.

Hardcastle WJ, 'New Methods of Profiling Lingual Palatal Contact Patterns with Electropalatography', *Work in Progress*, 4, p1, Phonetics Laboratory, University of Reading, 1984.

Hardcastle WJ, Morgan Barry R & Nunn M, 'Instrumental Articulatory Phonetics in Assessment and Remediation: Case Studies with the Electropalatograph', Stengelhofen J (ed), *Cleft Palate: The Nature and Remediation of Communication Problems*, Churchill Livingstone, Edinburgh, 1989.

Heinmann-de Boer JA, *Cleft Palate Children and Intelligence*, Swets & Zeitlinger, Lisse, 1985.

Huskie CF, 'The Glasgow Experience', Ellis RE & Flack FC (eds), *Diagnosis and Treatment of Palatoglossal Malfunction*, The College of Speech Therapists, London, 1979.

Huskie CF, 'Assessment of Speech and Language Status: Subjective and Objective Approaches to Appraisal of Vocal Tract Structure and Function', Stengelhofen J (ed), *Cleft Palate: The Nature and Remediation of Communication Problems*, Churchill Livingstone, Edinburgh, 1989.

Ingram D, *Phonological Disability in Children*, Edward Arnold, London, 1976.

Judson SL & Burden RL, 'Towards a Tailor-made Measure of Parental Attitudes. An Approach to the Evaluation of One Aspect of Intervention

Projects with Parents of Handicapped Children', *Child Care, Health and Development*, 6, p47, 1980.

Kaplan EN, 'The Occult Sub-mucous Cleft', *Cleft Palate Journal*, 12, p356, 1975.

Kernahan DA & Stark RB, 'A New Classification for Cleft Lip and Palate', *Plastic and Reconstructive Surgery*, 22, p435, 1958.

Klein MD, *Feeding Techniques for Children who have Cleft Lip and Palate*, Therapy Skill Builders, Communication Skill Builders, Tucson, Arizona, 1987.

Lancaster G & Pope L, *Working with Children's Phonology*, Winslow Press, Bicester, 1989.

McWilliams BJ, Morris HL & Shelton RL, *Cleft Palate Speech*, BC Decker Inc, Pennsylvania, 1984.

Martin S, *Working with Dysphonics*, Winslow Press, Bicester, 1988.

Masters FW, Bingham HG & Robinson DW, 'The prevention and Treatment of Hearing Loss in the Cleft Palate Child,' *Cleft Palate Journal*, 5, p44, 1960.

Morley M, *Cleft Palate Speech*, 7th edn, E & S Livingstone, Edinburgh, 1970.

Morris HJ, 'The Speech Pathologist Looks at the Tonsils and Adenoids, *Annals of Otology, Rhinology and Laryngology*', 84, p63, 1975.

Morris SE & Klein MD, *Pre-feeding Skills*, Therapy Skill Builders, Tucson, Arizona, 1987.

Paradise JL, 'Middle Ear Problems Associated with Cleft Palate,' *Cleft Palate Journal*, 12, p17, 1975.

Peterson HA, Marquardt TP & Thomas P, *Appraisal and Diagnosis of Speech and Language Disorders*, Prentice-Hall, New York, 1981.

Phillips P & Stengelhofen J, 'Towards Partnership with Parents', Stengelhofen J (ed), *Cleft Palate: The Nature and Remediation of Communication Problems*, Churchill Livingstone, Edinburgh, 1989.

Pigott R, 'Assessment of Velopharyngeal Function', Edwards M & Watson ACH (eds), *Advances in the Management of Cleft Palate*, Churchill Livingstone, Edinburgh, 1980.

Ruscello DM, St Louis KO, Barry P & Barry K, 'A Screening Method for the Evaluation of the Peripheral Speech Mechanism', *Folio Phoniatrica*, 34, 1982.

Russell J, 'Early Intervention', Stengelhofen J (ed), *Cleft Palate: The Nature and Remediation of Communication Problems*, Churchill Livingstone, Edinburgh, 1989.

Sell D & Woodard M, 'The Sri Lankan Cleft Lip and Palate Project', *Speech Therapy in Practice*, vol. 3, no. 1, June 1987.

Selley WG, 'Dental and Technical Aids for the Treatment of Patients Suffering from Velopharyngeal Disorders', Ellis RE & Flack FC (eds), *Diagnosis and Treatment of Palatoglossal Malfunction*, The College of Speech Therapists, London, 1979.

Shprintzen RJ, 'Velopharyngeal Insufficiency in the Absence of Overt or Submucous Cleft Palate: The Mystery Solved', Ellis RE & Flack FC (eds), *Diagnosis and Treatment of Palatoglossal Malfunction*, The College of Speech Therapists, London, 1979.

Spriestersbach DC, *Psychological Aspects of the 'Cleft Palate Problem'*, University of Iowa Press, Iowa, 1973.

Stengelhofen J (ed), *Cleft Palate: The Nature and Remediation of Communication Problems*, Churchill Livingstone, Edinburgh, 1989.

Stengelhofen J & Foster TD, 'An Investigation into the Effects of Residual Oro-nasal Fistula in Repaired Cleft Palate', *Proceedings of the 8th National Conference of the College of Speech Therapists*, London, 1979.

Stuffins GM, 'The Use of Appliances in the Treatment of Speech Problems in Cleft Palate', Stengelhofen J (ed), *Cleft Palate: The Nature and Remediation of Communication Problems*, Churchill Livingstone, Edinburgh, 1989.

Sweeny K, 'Personal Communication: experiences from VSO Fiji project', 1989.

Taberham J & Ball O, *Best Ever Minimal Pairs Pictures*, IMP Publishing Company/Winslow Press, Bicester, 1987.

Templin ML & Darley FL, *Templin–Darley Test of Articulation*, University of Iowa Press, Iowa, 1969.

Travis EL (ed), *Handbook of Audiology and Speech Pathology*, Appleton Century Crofts, New York, 1971.

Tudor C & Selley WG, 'A Palatal Training Appliance and a Visual Speech Aid for Use in the Treatment of Hypernasal Speech', *British Journal of Disorders of Communication*, 9, p2, 1974.

Van Demark DR, 'The Trouble with Speech Pathology. Letters to the Editor', *Cleft Palate Journal*, 20, p1, 1983.

Van Demark DR & Hardin MA, 'Effectiveness of Intensive Articulation Therapy for Children with Cleft Palate', *Cleft Palate Journal*, 23, p3, 1986.

Weiss CE, Lillywhite HS & Gordon ME, *Clinical Management of Articulation Disorders*, CV Mosby & Co, St Louis, 1980.

Wells CG, *Cleft Palate and its Associated Disorders*, McGraw Hill, New York, 1971.

Wilson DK, *Voice Problems of Children*, 3rd edn, Williams & Wilkins, Baltimore, 1987.

Witzel MA, Tobe J & Salyer KE, 'The Use of Videonasopharyngoscopy for Biofeedback Therapy in Adults after Pharyngeal Flap Surgery', *Cleft Palate Journal*, 26, 2, pp129–135, 1989.